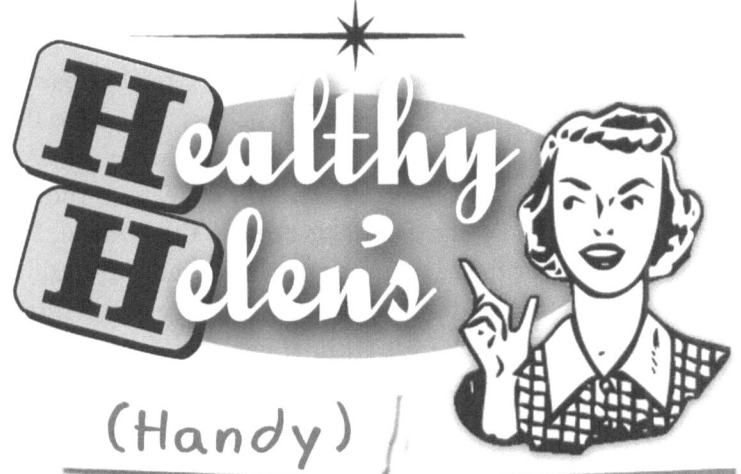

Healthy Helen's

(Handy)

HANDBOOK

OF FUNKY & FUNCTIONAL FOODSTUFFS

Dear Reader and Food Fan:

Welcome the wonderful world of functional foods!

Of course, you may not be a newcomer to this parallel world, but a long-time resident; maybe less a food fan than a full-fledged fanatic. Perhaps, like me, you're simply fascinated by food — where it's grown, how it's picked, produced or processed, and what its effects are, on the body and the planet. Whatever the case, my hope is that you will find this book educational, entertaining, and maybe even inspiring in your ongoing odyssey for optimal health and happiness.

Speaking of inspiration, this book was originally created as a compilation of entries first published in a weekly column called "Marge's Menu," which appeared in a Midwestern newspaper, *The Octopus*. Since that time, the paper has folded, I've moved to San Francisco, Marge has been given a makeover, and the compilation has been re-designed and updated with a bunch of newfound, newfangled foods.

A couple caveats: since the info in this book was gleaned from thousands of websites, many of which may be defunct, I have not bothered to list my sources (except for photo credits). If you are troubled by the bits of inaccurate or outdated information you might encounter, I'm always happy to be contacted and corrected, Also, and importantly, despite the prevalence of exotic items featured herein, I encourage everyone to buy local, organic food when possible, and/or grow it yourself. It's the healthy way to go!

With warmth,

Healthy Helen

(aka Darrin Drda*)

MAIN MENU

Although alphabetized in the book, the following foods have also been categorized for you convenience.

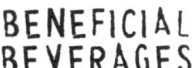

BENEFICIAL BEVERAGES

Green Tea
Guarana
Kombucha
Rooibos
Yerba Mate

FRIENDLY FRUITS & VEGGIES

Acai
Asafoetida
Bok Choy
Celeriac
Chile Peppers
Fiddlehead Ferns
Garlic
Goji Berries
Jerusalem Artichoke
Kale
Kiwifruit
Kohlrabi
Maca
Mangosteen
Noni
Okra
Plantains
Pomegranate
Pumpkin
Rapini
Sorrel
Sprouts
Tomato
Umeboshi

GREAT GRAINS

Alfalfa
Amaranth
Barley
Basmati Rice
Blue Corn
Brown Rice
Buckwheat
Job's Tears
Kamut
Millet
Quinoa
Sorghum
Spelt
Teff
Triticale
Wild Rice

HELPFUL HERBS

Ashwagandha
Asparagus Root
Astragalus
Bamboo Manna
Bhringaraj
Boswellia
Cat's Claw

Damiana
DongQuai
Epazote
Fennel
Fo-Ti
Gingko
Gotu Kola
Holy Basil
Kava Kava
Ma Huang
Marsh Mallow
Nettle
Oregano
Parsley
PauD'arco
St.John's Wort
Sarsaparilla
Schizandra
Shilajit
Yarrow

LOVELY LEGUMES
Adzuki Beans
Chick Peas
Fava Beans
Lentils
Lupins
Mung Beans
Pigeon Peas
Winged Beans

MIGHTY MUSHROOMS
Maitake
Reishi
Shiitake
Yamabushitake

OILS & SEEDS
Flax Seeds
Grapeseed Oil
Grapeseeds
Hemp Seeds
Primrose Oil
Rice Bran Oil
Sesame Oil
Tea Tree Oil
Wild Celery Seeds

SOY FOODS
Miso
Natto
Okara & Yuba
Seitan
Tamari, Shoyu
Tempeh
Textured Soy Protein

SPECIAL SPICES
Cayenne
Saffron
Sage
Thyme
Turmeric

HELPFUL KELP
Arame
Carrageen
Dulse, Wakame, Hijiki
Kombu
Kanten
Nori

SUBTERRANEAN SUSTENANCE

Burdock
Daikon
Galangal
Ginger
Ginseng
Jicama
Kuzu
Licorice Root
Lotus Root
Suma
Sweetpotato
Taro

SUPERFOODS

Aloe Vera Juice
Apple Cider Vinegar
Barley Grass
Broccoli Sprouts
Chlorella
Dunaliella
Royal Jelly
Spirulina
Wheatgrass Juice

SWEET SOMETHINGS

Agave Nectar
Amazake
Cacao
Carob
Mochi
Molasses
Stevia
Sucanat
Yacon

OTHER ODDITIES

Acidophilus
Balsamic Vinegar
Brewer's Yeast
Colostrum
Hominy
Nutritional Yeast
Psyllium
Tahini, Sesame Products
Wasabi
Wheat Germ

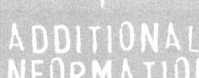

ADDITIONAL INFORMATION

ACAI

(pronounced "ah-sigh-EE") is a small, dark purple berry that grows on the Acai Palm, which grows in the Amazon rainforest of Brazil. Although diminutive in size and full of inedible seeds, acai has an impressive nutritional profile that has led to its being called "the world's #1 superfood" by a certain Dr. Perricone and by an equally certain Oprah Winfrey. More tentatively, the *NY Times* has called acai "one of the most nutritional fruits of the Amazon." Any way you pick it, acai packs more antioxidant power than any other fruit (ten times that of grapes), contains an abundance of amino acids and protein (almost 8% by weight), minerals like calcium, magnesium, potassium, and zinc, as well as Vitamins A, B1, B2, B3, E, and as much Vitamin C as blueberries. For a fruit, acai is also uncommonly full of fiber (14%) and fat (almost 50%, with most of that being of the healthy, unsaturated variety like Omega 3, 6, and 9). Because of their fattiness, acai berries tend to go rancid soon after being picked, and thus their pulp must be frozen or freeze-dried in order to be exported. Fortunately, a number of companies have been doing just that for the last decade or so, during which time acai has been gaining in popularity the world over (especially in Hawaii and California). Even more fortunately, the most popular companies such as Earthfruits and Sambazon (Sustainable Management of the Brazilian Amazon) provide organic, fairly-traded, and sustainably-harvested acai for the benefit of not only the dwindling rainforest but its human inhabitants, who can now sell fruit instead of lumber. Of course, the benefits also extend to people like you and me, who get to eat this tasty superfruit in acai bowls (containing other fruits and granola), smoothies and health drinks.

ACIDOPHILUS

Your intestines are home to about 400 types of bacteria, which make up about 3 pounds of your total weight. The friendliest of these species is probably *Lactobacillus acidophilus*, which survives mainly off of lactose (milk sugar), as its first name suggests. By helping produce chemicals like acidophilin, a natural antibiotic more powerful than even penicillin, acidophilus fights harmful bacteria like *salmonella, e. coli, staphlococcus*, and *candide albicans*, which causes yeast infections. A shortage of acidophilus can lead to infection by these nasty germs, as well as to rheumatoid arthritis, herpes, diabetes, meningitis, or chronic fatigue syndrome. The number of good bacteria in your gut is lowered by poor diet, stress, antibiotics (which tend to wipe out both good and bad bacteria), or ingestion of red meat, which usually contains the antibiotics and steroids often fed to cattle. In addition to killing bad bacteria, acidophilus helps make B vitamins, which tend to get destroyed by sugar, processed foods, coffee, birth control pills, and those darned antibiotics. Acidophilus also aids in protein digestion, prevents diarrhea and constipation, diminishes bad breath and B.O., and somehow even helps lower cholesterol. The acidophilus found in yogurt is not always active and is at a low concentration. The best way to get this helpful microorganism is in a pill. It comes in dairy-free form, but make sure to read the label. Brands that need to be refrigerated are unstable and get less potent over time.

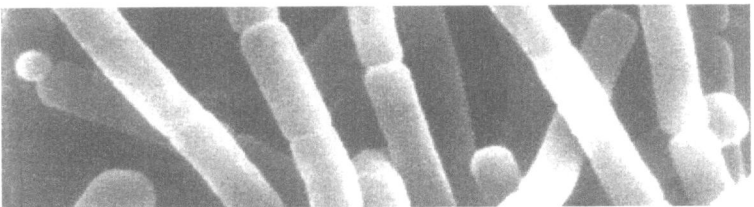

http://www.immunesupportonline.com

ADZUKI BEANS

Folks in Japan call them the "king of beans," though they're actually seeds from a bush-like plant from China and Korea that nowadays is grown in America and Europe as well. They're full of potassium and yummy yang energy that's good for your innards, especially your liver and kidneys, and can be put into pies, pizzas, patés, soups, served with vegetables and grains, or cooked with raisins to make a dessert. Azukis, as theyre also called, are small and hard but will get five times bigger when cooked. Like all legumes, they cook faster if soaked beforehand, preferably overnight. Dump out the old water and add 4 cups of new water for every cup of beans, and boil, with a little seaweed thrown in for good measure, for about an hour and 15 minutes. Then add a sprinkle of salt and soy, turn up the burner a bit, and boil for another 15 minutes or so until the beans are soft.

To make a side dish with pumpkin, add 2 cups of cubes and a sliced onion to your 1 cup of beans after they've boiled for 45 minutes, and continue the above process. If you're kidneys are ailing you, boil a couple tablespoons of beans in 8 cups of water, add a dash of tamari, and drink a little of the concoction thrice daily.

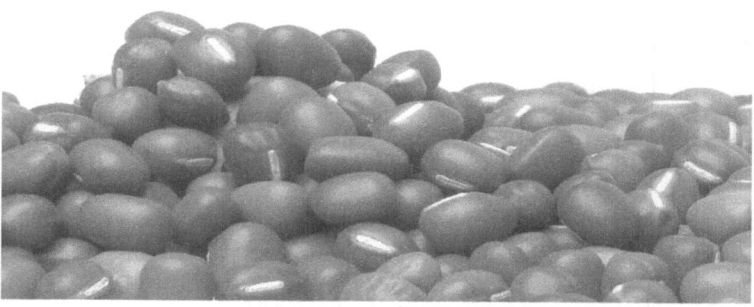

www.nutsonline.com

4

AGAVE NECTAR

This sticky substance is made from a cactus-like plant that bears a resemblance to yucca and a relationship to Aloe Vera. Although there are over 100 species of agave, the one most prized for production is Blue Agave, which is also used to make tequila. This is due to Blue Agave's high carbohydrate content, which yields a nectar high in fructose (the kind of sugar found in fruits). In Mexico, agave nectar is called *aguamiel* or "honey water," which hints at its consistency and at its use as a healthy alternative to the gooey stuff made by unpaid insects. Interestingly, the way bees make honey is similar to the way agave plants make nectar — by breaking down complex sugars into simple ones through the addition of enzymes. But unlike honey, agave nectar is low in glucose and high in natural fructose (as opposed to the processed kind made from corn). Also, agave nectar is sweeter than honey or table sugar, meaning that less is required. In baking recipes, for example, 1/3 - 3/4 cup agave nectar can be substituted for one cup of sugar, and the the baking temperature can by lowered by about 25 degrees, thereby saving energy too. Agave nectar comes in light and dark varieties, the former of which tastes a tad like maple syrup.

The agave plant

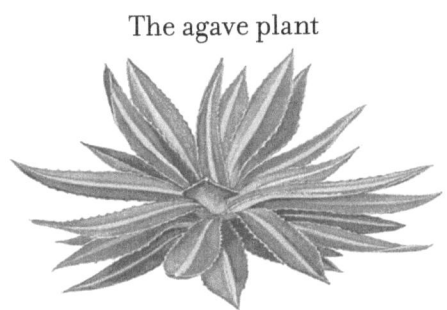

http://aggie-horticulture.tamu.edu

ALFALFA

This plant is probably native to Asia Minor, where its name originated. To Arabs, who long ago noticed that alfalfa made their horses fast and strong, "Al" refers to Allah, and "falf" means "the father of foods." The first documented use of alfalfa as a curative herb was in China, where it handled such ailments as swelling and kidney stones. It wasn't until the middle of last century that alfalfa began being cultivated in America, and nowadays about 20 million US acres are devoted to alfalfa, a crop which accounts for around 60% of the hay in the USA. A horse, of course, may say "hooray," but I say "nay," as alfalfa is good for humans, too. Fortunately, it is becoming more popular in its dried, powdered form, which packs a nutritional wollup. Two tablespoons of the stuff has twice as much calcium as milk, as much protein as a burger, as much iron as two ounces of liver, as well as B vitamins, fiber to help lower cholesterol, minerals like potassium, magnesium, and phosphorus, and enzymes aplenty. Another of alfalfa's charms is that it may have the highest chlorophyll content of any food. Chlorophyll, particularly abundant in sprouted grasses, is a great blood purifier and natural deodorant. In addition to its encapsulated form, alfalfa is sold as an earthy-tasting tea or as an extract, which, unfortunately, usually contains alcohol that can decrease its potency.

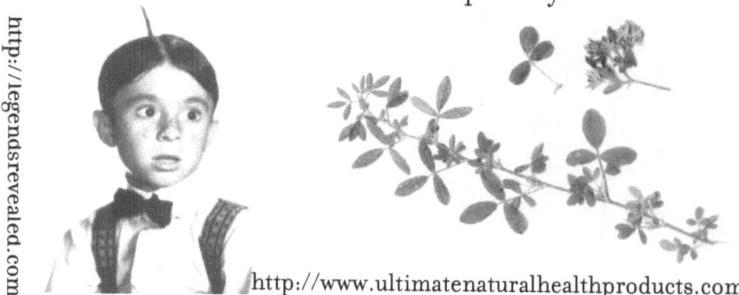

ALOE VERA JUICE

There are over 2000 varieties of the aloe plant, ranging in size from one measly inch to as tall as a tree. The most familiar and beneficial type is definitely *barbadensis miller*, a.k.a. aloe vera, or "the true aloe." This cactus-like desert plant, actually a relative of onion and garlic, has been used for healing purposes since ancient Greek, Hebrew, and Egyptian times, by such notable non-healers as Alexander the Great and Columbus. It's been called "the medicine plant" by the Chinese, "the miracle plant that heals itself" by native Americans, and "the burn plant" by Africans. Modern Americans are probably most familiar with its ability to help heal wounds and moisturize skin, but aloe vera has tradition-ally been used in other countries to make a curative beverage and laxative. Its chubby leaves, made up of 3 layers including the inner, active gel layer, can be pressed and filtered to make a juice that supposedly contains 7 of the 8 essential aminos, vitamins A, B_1, B_2, B_6, B_{12}, C and E, minerals like magne-sium, calcium, iron, potassium, and zinc, as well as enzymes aplenty to enhance the absorption of these nutrients. This juice has been used effectively against peptic ulcers, arthri-tis, and diabetes, and to upgrade the immune system in gen-eral. It been shown to reverse feline leukemia, and is being investigated as a treatment for HIV, as it contains a chemical called acemannan that seems to greatly enchance the effects of the drug AZT. If you're buying aloe vera juice, check the label carefully. A cheap price might mean a low concentrate; "100% pure" could (legally) refer to a little juice mixed with a lot of water. Also, make sure the stuff is cold-pressed, as heat can destroy nutrients. The recommended dose is from 2-4 ounces per day, either straight or mixed with fruit juice.

AMARANTH

There are about 60 species of *Amaranthus*, most of which first grew in the Americas. The ancient peoples of this region ate as much of the grain as they did maize. They also used the seeds, which pop like popcorn when heated up, in religious rituals (the Spanish invaders were upset by this and tried to eradicate the stuff). Nowadays, amaranth is cultivated for its grain (which isn't technically a grain at all, but looks and cooks like one), its greens (which are sometimes purplish or red), and its pretty, little flowers (which grow in pink, dark red, or purple clusters at the top). Most varieties grow wild and are edible, but not so tasty. Amaranth grain, *Amaranthus edulis*, has more calcium, iron, potassium, phosphorus, and magnesium than any other grain (it's got 5 times the iron of wheat, and 3 times the fiber). It also rules protein-wise, at about 16%. Better yet, the protein is of a superior quality, containing lots of Lysine, a body- and brain-building amino acid that's hard to come by in other grains. Amaranth greens are similarly high in protein, calcium (twice as much as milk) and iron. Another great thing about Amaranth is that it's easy to grow and uses a minimal amount of water. It seems to grow like mad in soil that is otherwise unusable. Use a little more water than grain when cooking. When mixed with other grains like wheat, corn, or brown rice, it provides as much complete protein as meat. It can also be put into soup or porridge, and makes one heck of a pancake mix.

AMAZAKE

(or amasaki) is a sweet rice ferment made from brown rice and *koji*. Koji, a cute little fungus also used to make soy, tamari, and sake, causes enzymes to break down the rice's proteins and starches into simpler sugars. This results in a naturally sweet, pudding-like substance which is usually then blended and strained into a milky consistency and sold as a drink. It can be frozen into tasty popsicles, blended with fruit and a little water to make smoothies, or used instead of milk to sweeten and moisten bread or cookie recipes (although, in baking, it's not quite sweet enough to do the trick by itself). You can buy amasake in health food stores, or make your own if you happen to have some koji lying around:

Boil 1 cup of brown rice in 4 cups of water amd simmer for an hour or so, until the water is gone. In a ceramic or glass bowl, mix the rice with 1 cup of sweet brown rice koji, 1 cup of warm water, and a pinch of salt. Cover and incubate at about 95°, either on a hot plate, in a very low oven, or in a sauna (if you have one of those lying around). After 6 or 8 hours, add a little more water and boil again for a few minutes.

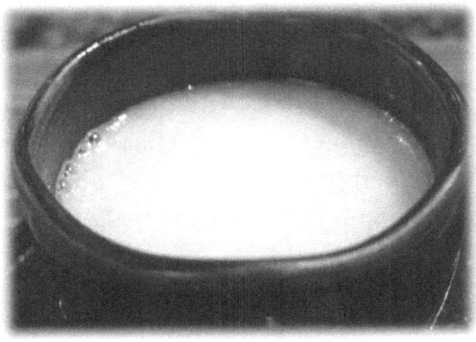

http://kimoto.cc

9

APPLE CIDER VINEGAR

The dictionary defines vinegar as "a sour liquid obtained by acetic fermentation of dilute ethyl alcoholic liquids," which, in English, means that it comes from drinks like wine and cider that have been sitting around for a while. Ye olde French method takes about 5 or six months, but nowadays we have machines and heat which speed up the fermentation process but lower the nutritional value. The benefits of cider vinegar have been known since Bible times. Later, in Greek times, Hippocrates (Mr. Medicine himself) prescribed it to his patients for its natural antibiotic and antiseptic properties. It has a lot of potassium, helps regulate calcium metabolism and menstruation, helps the digestive system do its thing, and helps to keep the blood flowing smoothly by flushing out toxins and dissolving acid crystals that build up in the joints and cause stiffness and arthritis. It's good for the bones, the skin, the sinuses, and soothes sore throats and sunburns. Folklore says that it can be taken by a pregnant female to insure a male baby. A doctor named Gabe Cousens, who wrote a book called *Conscious Eating*, says "Apple cider vinegar is the #1 food that I recommend for maintaining the body's vital acid-alkaline balance." Another fella named Paul Bragg, who calls himself a "Life Extension Specialist," calls apple cider vinegar "a miracle" and wrote a whole book about it. He says 1-2 teaspoons daily with the same amount of honey helps humans live longer and keeps fleas off of his pigs. Cider vinegar is often seen in salad dressings and can be combined with molasses, pepper and tamari to make a BBQ sauce.

ARAME

Sea vegetables, among the Earth's most ancient life forms and maybe the oldest foodstuffs harvested by humans, are a remarkable source of nutrition, packing some 13 vitamins, including A, B, C, and D, 20 amino acids, and 60 trace elements like calcium, iron, and iodine. Arame is a brown kind of seaweed used most commonly in Japanese cooking. Its large leaves are harvested, dried, then shredded into delicate, spaghetti-like ribbons that cook up in a jiffy after a few minutes of presoaking. It's got protein, lots of calcium, potassium, and iodine, and a flavor that's not fishy, but mild, almost sweet.

To make an exotic, aquatic side dish, simmer arame with tamari and either lemon juice, ginger and garlic, or vinegar and barley malt, then sprinkle with sesame seeds. Sautée it with tofu, or add it to stir fries, noodle dishes, or miso-based soups.

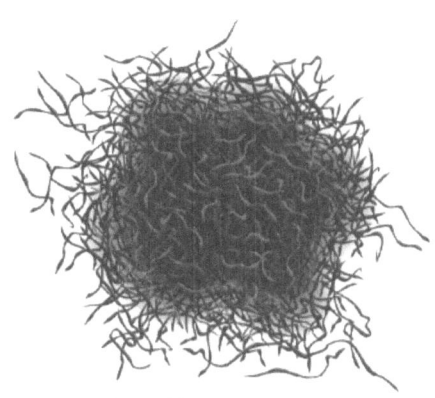

http://img.quamut.com

ASAFOETIDA

Sometimes spelled without the "o," this tall perennial from the parsley family is native to the Middle East, where its cabbage-like leaves are eaten raw by people and animals alike. The herb's Latin name, *Ferula foetida* (meaning "fetid sap"), and the nickname "devil's dung" both refer to the stinky, reddish resin that oozes from the roots of mature plants when cut. This gummy substance contains natural sulfur compounds similar to those found in onions and garlic, for which asafoetida is sometimes substituted in cooking. In Traditional Chinese Medicine, asafeotida is thought to stimulate the respiratory, intestinal and nervous systems and benefit the stomach, liver and spleen, while in Ayurveda, "hing" is classified as *pitta* or "fiery," and is used against bronchitis, pneumonia, hysteria, intestinal parasites, and flatulence. The resin is sold in small lumps, or as a powder or paste that often winds up in curries, spicy pickles, lentil dishes (dahl), or in a rejuvenating concoction called "hingashtak," which also includes ginger, cumin, salt, peppers, and other herbs. Asafoetida, which is also called "narthex," contains calcium, phosphorus, iron, and some of the B vitamins.

Asafoetida resin

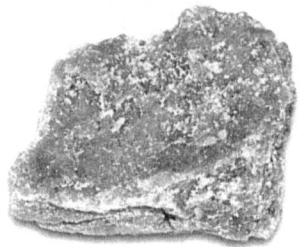

aidanbrooksspices.blogspot.com

ASPARAGUS ROOT

The Persian word *asparag*, which means something like "edible shoot," actually comes from ancient Greece, when and where wild asparagus was consumed as a veggie and as a remedy for insect bites, toothaches, and heart problems. A favorite of Louis XIV, asparagus spears (which incidentally can grow up to 10 inches per day) have been used over the ages to treat kidney, liver, and stomach problems, memory loss, tuberculosis, and sexual disorders, while their slender shape has earned them a reputation as an aphrodesiac. Nutritionally, asparagus has been found to contain antitumor chemicals called saponins, not to mention plenty of good old fiber, potassium, and vitamins A, C, B2, and B6. Anyhow, apart from the garden variety, *Asparagus officinalis*, another important species is *A. racemosus*, known as "asparagus root" since that's the part that gets eaten. While regular asparagus originated in southern Europe, this plant is native to India, where it's called *shatavari*, meaning "possessor of 100 husbands." As you might guess, the herb is used in Ayurveda to pump up fertility and rejuvenate the female organs, although it can be consumed by both genders to strengthen the blood and nurture the mucous membranes, as well as to treat most of the maladies mentioned above. Overall, the energy of the plant is said to be *saatvic*, increasing love, devotion, and peace of mind. Asparagus root is usually dried, ground, and taken with milk and sugar; otherwise it's made into a paste that can also be used externally on aching joints and muscles.

ASTRAGALUS

This herb comes from the root of *astragalus membranaceus*, a perennial legume that grows wild in Mongolia and northern China, where it's been used since ancient times to strengthen "wei ch'i (qi)" or "defensive energy," what Westerners might call the immune system. Modern Chinese doctors give "huang qi" to people undergoing chemotherapy, and studies confirm that these patients do show a stronger immunity and higher survival rate than those who don't ingest the herb. It also protects bone marrow, which tends to get deteriorated from radiation. Astragalus is also commonly used to combat colds, flu, respiratory problems, and stress-related conditions, and has antibacterial properties. Its power lies mostly in its bioflavenoids and polysaccharides (especially one called "astragalan B"), and partly in its concentrations of the B vitamin choline and the mineral selenium. The American version of astragalus is called "milk vetch root" or "yellow emperor." In some species, such as the one known as "locoweed" in the Old West, the above-ground parts can make animals who eat them sick, or at least cause them to act goofy. For humans, astragalus is available dried, in capsules, or as an extract. In China, the root is often sold in bundles of popsicle-stick-shaped slices, which are dropped into teas and soups, or pan-fried with honey.

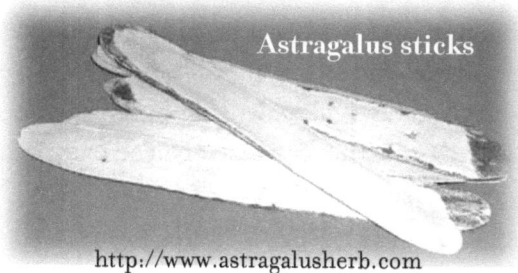

Astragalus sticks

http://www.astragalusherb.com

BALSAMIC VINEGAR

The authentic version of this fancy foodstuff comes from Modena, Italy, hometown of Luciano Pavarotti. It was there, in 1598, that the vinegar-loving Duke of Este set up a unique industry that continues to this day. The traditional brewing method, which predates both The Voice and the Duke, involves pressing sweet *Trebbiano* grapes into a pulpy liquid or "must" (*saba* to Italians), which gets simmered in copper kettles for a day or so, filtered, then fermented in a *batteria* of old barrels made from oak, ash, juniper, chestnut, cherry, and mulberry woods, each contributing their subtle flavors to the final product. Italian law states that *Balsamico Tradizionale* must be aged for at least 12 years, although certain producers will let it sit around for 30, 50 or even 100 years, resulting in a concoction so flavorful that it's often sipped after dinner like port wine. Classified in Italy as a "food" rather than a "vinegar," true "artisan" quality balsamic comes in short, rectangular bottles labeled with the seal of the "Consortio ABTM," an elite group of traditional Modena producers. As you can imagine, the stuff can get pretty pricey, going for as much as $100 per ounce. The cheaper, industrial-grade *aceto balsamico* that most people buy is usually some type of wine vinegar, sometimes containing sugar, caramel coloring, and licorice or vanilla flavoring. Although more acidic than the real thing, it's perfectly suitable for everyday use, adding its well-balanced sweet-sour flavor to soups, sauces, and stews. It also tastes great straight, sprinkled on salad or fresh fruit. Like other vinegars, balsamic aids digestion and helps break down fat and cholesterol.

BAMBOO MANNA

With root systems categorized as either "runners" (more common in temperate varieties) or "clumpers" (consolidated in the tropics), bamboo is a type of wild grass whose stems or "culms" can be as thick as 30cm in diameter and as much as 30m tall. Increasing in height by up to 4 feet per day in one species, bamboo has the distinction of being the fastest-growing plant on the planet. It is also one of the most vigorous, as evidenced by groves near ground zero in Hiroshima which remained standing after the atomic blast or grew back within days. Long revered in the Orient for both its elegant beauty and practical value, bamboo was also important to the Cherokee and Seminole peoples of southeastern North America, where the plant was once common. While being used to make things like boats, buildings, furniture, and paper, bamboo also has a traditional use as a food and medicine. In both Traditional Chinese Medicine and Ayurveda, the species *bambusa arundinaceae* is valued for its leaves and its milky inner bark, called "bamboo manna." Known as "Zhu ru" in China and "vamsha rochana" in India, this substance is thought to have rejuvenating and moisturizing effects on the lungs, a soothing effect on the nerves, and a fortifying effect on the blood. While being generally strengthening and nourishing, its primary application is to ease fever, coughs, and other symptoms of colds and flu. In fact, bamboo manna is a primary ingredient in an Ayurvedic anti-cold formula called "sito paladi" that also contains ginger, cinnamon, cardamom, pippali (Indian pepper), and sugar, which helps the medicine go down.

BARLEY,

a relative of rice, may be the planet's oldest cultivated grain, first cropping up in Mesopotamia in 8,000 BCE or so. Egyptians living around 4500 BCE ate it, as did Sumerians, who used bags of the stuff as currency, and it gets mentioned in the Bible. It ruled Europe, too, until dethroned by wheat and rye in the Middle Ages. Today, it's one of the most important foods for Tibetans, and in Scotland it's an indispensible ingredient in beer, whiskey and gin. It's also big in Japan, where "mugi" often gets roasted and boiled to make "mugicha" tea, or fermented to make miso. Here in the States, barley is used mostly as animal food and to make booze, which is too bad, as it's quite nutritious, with gobs of fiber to keep you regular, as well as chemicals like "glucan" to lower cholesterol and "hordenine" to help with circulation. Plus, it's lower in fat than most grains. "Pearled" barley, by the way, refers to grains that have had their bran partially polished off. To prepare barley, soak the grains overnight and boil one cup with 4 or 5 cups of water for about 1-1/2 hours. Cooked, it can be used in salads, added to soups (it's especially yummy in split pea) or sautéed with mushrooms and veggies in broth. Barley is also sometimes germinated and heated into barley malt, a sweet syrup that contains protein, minerals, and complex sugars like maltose and dextrose that are more user-friendly than the simple sugars found in other sweeteners.

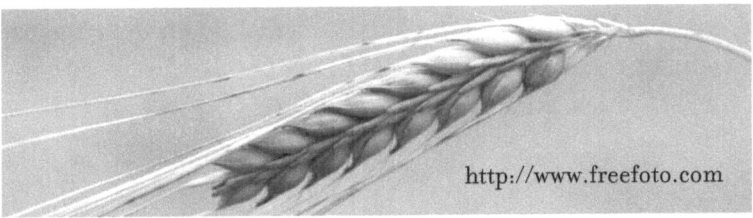

http://www.freefoto.com

BARLEY GRASS

The hardy barley plant has been cultivated in climates ranging from the tropics to the Arctic circle. Its main use has been as a grain, and as such, it's no nutritional slouch (see BARLEY). Where barley really packs a punch, however, is in its young grass stage. If picked when the plant is about a foot tall, the leaves are said to contain all the nutrition a human could ever need: 16 vitamins, 23 minerals, 18 of 20 bodily amino acids (including all 8 of the essentials), more detoxifying chlorophyll than even wheatgrass, and an abundance of enzymes, including "supper oxide dismutase," which has anti-aging powers. The powder usually made from barley grass juice supposedly has, by weight, 11 times the calcium of milk, 7 times the vitamin C of oranges, 5 times the iron of spinach, and double the protein of ground beef, as well as most of the B vitamins (especially B6 and B12), antioxidants including one more powerful than vitamin E, and a natural progesterone shown to slow and even reverse the effects of osteoporosis. Another great property of barley grass is its high alkalinity, which counteracts the high Ph levels found in most modern foods that make the body more vulnerable to illness and allergies. The most famous brand of concentrated barley grass is called "Barleygreen," created by Dr. Yoshihide Hagiwara, who once owned the biggest pharmaceutical company in Japan until mercury poisoning made him start losing his teeth, hair and skin. He then began studying leafy green foods and eventually found barley grass to have the most complete nutritional benefits. Today Dr. Hagiwara is happier, healthier, and probably pretty rich.

BASMATI RICE

Rice, called the "life-giving seed" in old Sanskrit books, is the staple food which directly feeds the most humans (without being first fed to animals). It's been cultivated for around 7,000 years; at first from swamps where it grew wild, then from human-flooded paddies, which were invented about 5,000 years back by the Chinese. Today there are about 7,000 varieties of this grain, most of them grown and eaten in Asia. One of the most famous, and certainly most distinctive-smelling types is basmati, whose name means "queen of fragrance." In India, the sweet, nutty aroma was thought to be a gift from the god Veda, although modern scientists (with more book learning and less imagination) now know that it comes from a certain chemical that's actually present in all rice. Most basmati is, in fact, grown in India (mostly in the Himalayan foothills), and in neighboring Pakistan. Most of what's sold in the US is an aromatic variety related to basmati, or a cross-breed called "Texmati." Like all rice types, basmati comes in white or brown; the former a bit more aromatic, the latter more nutritious, containing the bran that holds B vitamins, protein, and minerals like potassium. Both types are said to be easy to digest.

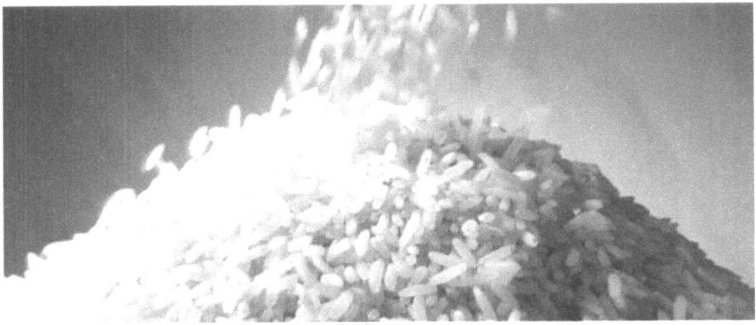

http://globalvisiongrp.com

BHRINGARAJ

Growing in the Himalayan foothills and along lakes and marshes in India as well as in the southwestern United States, this evergreen comes in white-flowering, yellow-flowering, and black-fruiting varieties, all of which are valued in Ayurveda for their ability to fight the effects of aging on the eyes, ears, bones, teeth and especially the hair. In fact, the herb's Hindi name (bhringaraj) and Sanskrit name, *keshraja*, both mean "ruler of the hair," as the juice of its leaves, often combined with coconut and sesame oils, is spread on the head to restore the darkness and luster of old follicles and promote the growth of new. Spread on the skin, the juice of *Ecliptica albans* is thought to improve the complexion, reduce inflammation, relieve joint pain, and help heal cuts and bruises. Taken internally, it is used against hepatitis, fever, congestion, and jaundice, which it can reportedly cure in less than a week. One of the celebrated qualities of bhringaraj, actually, is its beneficial effect on the liver, which can likewise be derived from its roots. Also touted are the plant's effects on the brain, which include improved memory, relief from headaches, a calming of the mind, and the promotion of restful sleep. The active ingredients in bhringaraj have been found to be an alkaloid called "ecliptine," and glucoside, which seems to have antiviral properties.

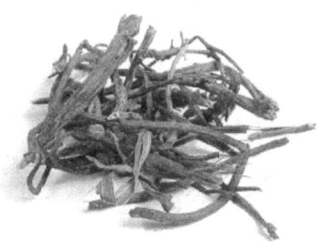

http://www.organicindia.com

BLUE CORN

Maize has been an important food in the Americas since forever. Mayas and Incas from south of the border used to worship the grain, believing that the first person was made from masa dough. Before Europeans became obsessed with white and yellow (dent) varieties, the main grain was blue corn, prized by Pueblos and considered by Hopi men to be a special source of strength. It's still fairly popular in the southwest, where it's used in foods like piki, a kind of thin bread, chaquegue, a cornmeal mush, and atole, a concoction often drank for breakfast with cinnamon and sugar. Northerners see this type of corn mostly in flakes, chips, and tortillas. Blue corn is a much more complete source of protein than its paler relatives, is higher in zinc and iron, and contains a natural starch that can be absorbed by the skin (certain companies sell a mixture that supposedly hydrates the face and releases toxins). Blue corn flour is more course and grainy than other kinds. In general, stone ground flours retain most of the hull, so they have more fiber, calcium, potassium, and other goodies than degermed flour, but also more oil, so they have to be kept in the fridge.

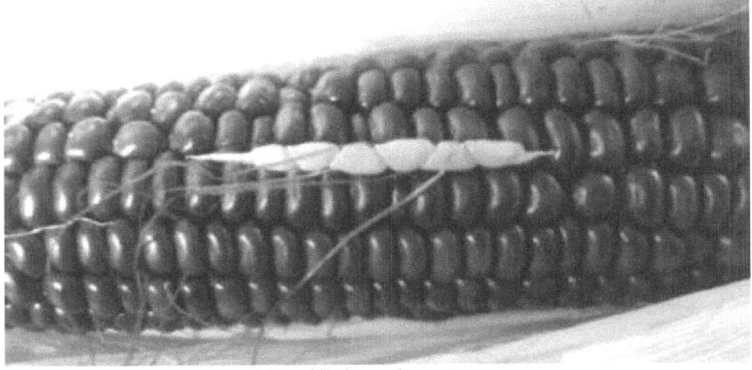

http://hila.webcentre.ca

BOK CHOY

(or baak choi), is a member of the mustard family. It's related to cabbage, its stalks look like celery and its dark green leaves look like chard, so it's also called Chinese Chard, Chinese (White or Mustard) Cabbage, or sometimes Chinese Celery. It's one of the most popular veggies in the Philippines, where it's called "pechay" or "petsai." In Korea, it's pickled with other vegetables to make the notorious kimchi (or kim chee). A variety called baby bok choy (or Shanghai bok choy or Ming Qing Choi or choy sum) is, as you might guess, smaller, with bright white stalks and spinachy leaves. Anyhow, no matter how you slice it or what you call it, brassica chinensis has no fat or cholesterol, almost no sodium or calories, and is a good source of vitamins A, B6, and C, and calcium to boot. Along with broccoli, brussel sprouts, cauliflower, and a bunch of other stuff that mom made you to eat, it's a cruciferous vegetable, containing special "phytochemicals" (*phyto* is Greek for "plant") that are being shown to fight cancer. When steaming or stir-frying in garlic and oil, cut the stalks diagonally, and shred the leaves or cut them into squares and add them later, since they cook even faster than the stalks.

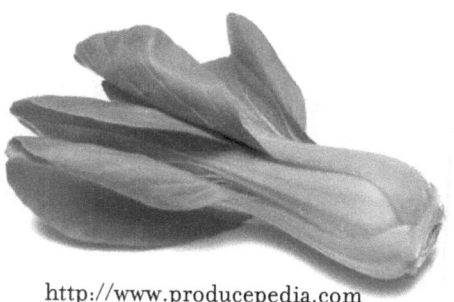

http://www.producepedia.com

BOSWELLIA

The large-branching tree from which this functional food comes grows mostly in dry, hilly areas of India, where its sap is called "salai guggal." In combination with other "guggals," or gummy resins, that of "Indian frankincense" has been used by Ayurvedic doctors for ages to treat diarrhea and dysentery in people, as well as inflammation in the joints of sacred cows. Modern scientists who've studied the effects of *Boswellia serrata* on humans have discovered that it does, indeed, seem to relieve the symptoms of rheumatism, gout, lower back pain, and arthritis. In fact, more and more doctors are prescribing Boswellia to arthritis sufferers as an alternative to aspirin, Ibuprofen, and other "non-steroidal anti-inflammatory drugs," whose side effects include kidney damage and ulcers. Boswellia is not only safe for the innards, but may actually help heal the type of gastrointestinal bleeding caused by these NSAIDs. Its magical ingredient, dubbed "boswellic acid," has been shown to increase circulation in the joints and inhibit the prostoglandins and leukotrines that cause painful, chronic swelling. In addition, Boswellia contains "circuminoids," antioxidants also present in turmeric which have proven themselves useful against cancer, heart disease, and respiratory disorders. Usually sold as an extract, Boswellia is not recommended for pregnant women or people with weakened immune systems.

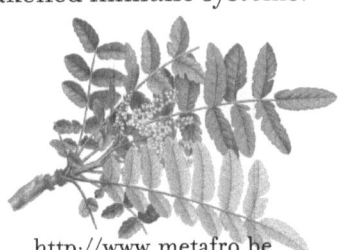

http://www.metafro.be

23

Yeasts are adorable little single-celled creatures who, lacking chlorophyll like the rest of the fungus family, must feast on other other beasts and plants to get their favorite food, oxygen. Yeast is useful in making ethanol for cars, bacterias for hepatitis and cancer research, and helping to clean up yukky stuff, like oil spills and waste material. The most common of the 160 or so species of yeast is called "*Saccharomyces cereviseae*" by people who insist on speaking Latin and "brewer's yeast" by us regular folks who like to get a little tipsy now and then. It is used in the making of booze to turn sugars and starches in grapes and grains into carbon dioxide and alcohol during fermentation. Brewer's yeast has loads of protein and B complex vitamins, so keep some in your cupboard even if you don't like liquor. One friend of mine pours it on top of popcorn, another puts it in her pet to make it extra healthy and fluffy.

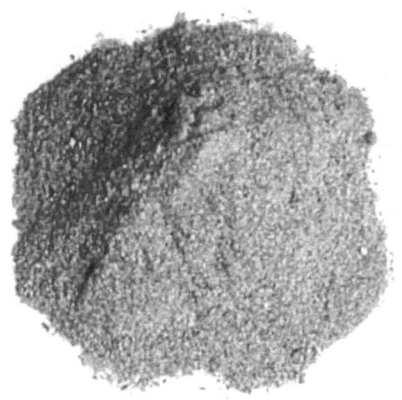

http://www.dkimages.com

BROCCOLI SPROUTS

A decade or so ago, scientists discovered that cruciferous veggies like cabbage, cauliflower, and kale contain chemicals called "isothiocyanates" that help fight cancer. In 1992, folks at Johns Hopkins University found that a particularly potent isothiocyanate called sulforaphane, which mobilizes anti-cancer enzymes and prevents tumors, was especially abundant in baby broccoli plants. In fact, at three days old, broccoli sprouts apparently contain 30-50 times more sulforaphane than grown-up broccoli. This means that instead of eating 2 pounds of (adult) broccoli per week (a dosage shown to cut the risk of colon cancer in half), a person would only have to eat 1 ounce of sprouts to get the same anti-cancer power. This, of course, is no problem, given how light, tasty and zingy the little things are. They are also quite easy to grow, like so:

Put 4 tbsp seeds in a sterilized, 32-oz jar, rinse, and drain. Cover the seeds with about a cup of water, secure some mesh or cheesecloth around the mouth of the jar, and set it in a dark, warmish place (like under the sink) overnight. Rinse and drain the seeds a few times a day for a few days, storing the jar in the dark place, upside-down, at an angle. Once the sprouts get little leaves, let them into the light for a day or so. Eat 'em raw or in this Broccoli-Tofu Spread: Mash 8 oz tofu with 1 tbsp miso, 4 tbsp tahini, and 2 tbsp lemon juice, then fold in in 3/4 cup of chopped sprouts. Spread the mixture on your favorite multi-grain bread.

BROWN RICE

Historians say that rice was probably first grown in India about 3,000 BCE and was brought to China and then Japan, Indonesia, and other parts of the planet. Today about half the people in the world live mainly on this grain, which comes from the aquatic *Oryza sativa* plant. Rice is harvested (by hand, usually) and milled (by machine,usually) to rub off the outer husk. In the case of white rice, the brown bran is also removed, greatly reducing the nutritional value and leaving just the starchy part, which, to add insult to injury, is sometimes coated with talc and glucose to make it look shiny in the supermarket. Brown, or whole grain, rice, on the other, healthy hand, is high in protein (about 8% by volume), iron, calcium, and the B vitamins niacin, riboflavin, and especially thiamine, a chemical needed to metabolize carbohydrates, like those in the inside part of the rice (duh). Mr. Macrobiotic, George Oshawa, called brown rice "soul food," with the perfect balance of yin and yang energy, and recommended eating it often, especially when one feels stressed or depressed. In my book, whole, organically-grown grains are the greatest. To cook brown rice, put 1 cup in a pot with 3 cups water and a pinch of salt, boil vigorously for 5 to 10 minutes, then lower the heat and simmer for a half hour or so, until the water is gone. Rice is nice with a touch of tamari, or it can be baked, fried, refrigerated, and reheated for use in anything from soups to desserts, casseroles to sushi rolls.

BUCKWHEAT

comes from a rhubarb-related plant that most likely originated in central Asia and was brought east to China and Japan, where it's been popular for a few millennia, and west to Europe, some say by those crazy Crusaders. Folks in eastern Europe and Russia love the stuff and call it "kasha," while English people used to use it to feed farm animals and foul. Buckwheat is considered a grain, but, if you want to get technical, it's actually more like a small, hard nut. When ground, the groats make a flour which is also dark and heavy, and so is sometimes mixed with a little wheat or rice flour to lighten it up, and then used to make muffins and stuff, or, in Japan, to make linguini-like noodles called "soba," which are often seen in soups. Kasha's got a lot of iron and B vitamins, contains more protein than most grains and is loaded with lysine, an amino acid that most grains don't have. It also has something called "rutic acid," which is good for circulation and high blood pressure, and helps the lungs, bladder and kidneys do their thing.

Make a healthy and hearty pancake mix with 1/2 cup of each of the following: buckwheat flour, whole wheat flour, soy milk, and cold water. Add a sprinkle of salt, 1/2 tsp. cinnamon, and, if you want, an egg (free range if you care about karma). Pour a thin layer of batter into a pre-oiled pan and cook up a kashacake or ten.

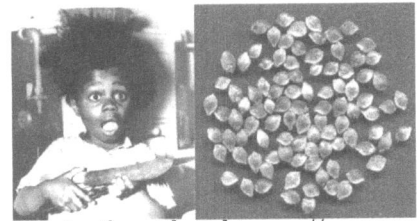

www.insignificantthoughts.com//www.vurv.cz

BURDOCK

is a bushy plant from the Sunflower family that grows, weedlike, mostly in Europe and the US. The Japanese call it "gobo," and are fond of its dark, slender root, although the whole plant is edible. The youngest of the big, waxy leaves, which give the plant the last part of its name, can be eaten as greens, while the stalks, removed before the purple flowers of *Arctium lappa* bloom in the spring, taste sort of like asparagus when boiled. The hooked seeds (fruit) inspired the creation of Velcro because of the way they stick like crazy to furry animals and clothing. When ground and eaten, they impart many of the same benefits as the root, which contains lots of a detoxifying carbohydrate called inulin, and is used to purify the blood, help digestion, treat ulcers, gout, arthritis, and rheumatism, and (on the outside of the body) skin diseases and hemmorrhoids. The Russians use burdock root to fight cancer, and Nicholas Culpepper, an old-time herbalist, wrote that it "helpeth those bit by a mad dog." Even if you're not sick or worried about nutty canines, the plant is a good source of iron and essential oils.

To make a flavorful side dish, whittle a scrubbed tuber into long chips, and do the same with a carrot or two. Sautée a chopped onion in a little oil, simmer it with the burdock and carrot sticks in a cup of vegetable stock for 20 minutes or so, then add a dash of toasted sesame oil or tamari for flavor.

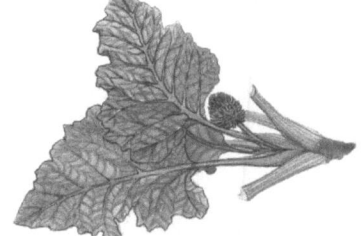

http://www.learningherbs.com

CACAO

Native to the Americas (most likely Amazonia), the cacao (cuh-KOW) or cocoa plant is a tropical evergreen whose nut-like seeds (usually called beans) are used to make chocolate in its various forms. It was named *cacahuatl* by the ancient Aztecs, imbibed medicinally and ritualistically by the Mayans, and used as a form of currency by many Mesoamerican cultures, right up until the 19th century. Even its scientific name, *Theobroma cacao*, means "food of the gods," indicating how revered it has been among foods. Of course, cacao is also used to make many earthly indulgences like candy bars and snack foods, which contain milk fat, sugar, artificial flavors, and other unhealthy stuff. On their own, however, cacao beans (which grow in clusters of 20-60) are actually good for you, with several times more antioxidants than green tea, a high percentage of monounsaturated (heart-healthy) fat, and minerals like magnesium, calcium, iron, sulfur, and zinc. Raw cacao is also a mood enhancer, containing a natural euphoric called anandamide, a natural aphrodesiac called arginine, a stimulant called theobromine, and a smidge of caffeine. Cacao beans are often dried, hulled and crushed into cacao nibs, which come either raw or roasted. Nibs are basically cacao in its purest form, with a taste more bitter than sweet, and can be used in baking recipes or eaten plain (sometimes combined with nuts, seeds, or dried berries like the goji). Dark chocolate is the next healthiest thing, the higher the percentage of cacao the better. Better yet is to buy cacao that's been organically grown and fairly traded.

Cacao pod with beans

http://www.cocoandme.com

CARDAMOM

Alternatively spelled "cardamum" or "cardamon," this "queen of spices" (black pepper being the king) comes from *Elettaria cardomomum*, a tropical relative of ginger whose flowering parts produce small, green pods filled with anywhere from 12 to 20 dark brown seeds. The pods are usually harvested by hand (a process which makes cardamom second only to saffron in price), then usually either kiln-dried to produce "green" cardamom or sun-dried to produce the less-coveted "black" cardamom (whose pods actually turn whitish). Sometimes called "grains of paradise," the seeds themselves have a strong smell and taste described as "pungent," "lemony," "flowery," or likened to anise or eucalyptus. Cardamom was supposedly a favorite of Cleopatra, who burned it to help seduce Marc Antony and others. It was also used by the Greeks and Romans, who imported it from India, where a good percentage of cardamom is still grown (other big producers are Sri Lanka and Guatemala). In Ayurvedic medicine, "ellaichi" (from which the plant's genus name is derived) is considered one of the best and safest digestive aids, helpful in ridding the body of gas and excess fluids (or "kapha") by stimulating the squeezing action of the intestines (parastalsis). It also works on the upper respiratory system to relieve coughs, colds, bronchitis, asthma, and hoarseness. In Indian cuisine, cardamom appears in the curries of the south and in the "garam masala" (hot spice) concoctions in the north, as well as being eaten after meals (usually pod and all, sometimes with fennel seeds) to aid digestion and to freshen the breath. Because of its ability to break down milk as well as detoxify caffeine, cardamom is often thrown into tea and coffee. In fact, 60% of the world's cardamom is consumed in the Middle East, mostly as an ingredient in Arabian coffee or "gahwa," which is usually drunk ritually (Bedouins consider it polite to slurp the beverage noisily). When brought to Europe in 1215, cardamom was considered an aphrodesiac, whereas nowadays its most common use in those parts is to flavor cakes, cookies, and other pastries. Although usually sold in its ground, powdery form, cardamom begins to lose its essential oils as soon as it's decorticated, or removed from the pod.

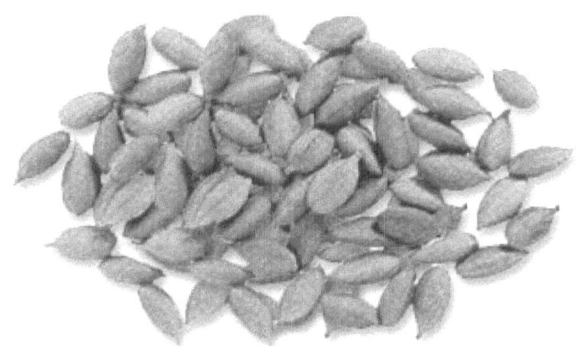

CAROB

is a type of bean with an edible, dark purple pod that comes from a leafy, green tree in the locust family. It is also called "St. John's bread" after the fella who baptized Jesus. The Bible says that he lived in the wilderness and ate honey and "locusts," but it means beans, not bugs, thank goodness. This legume has been consumed by critters and human people (saints and non-saints) for thousands of years, but has become popular in the last decade or so as a substitute for chocolate, which naturally contains caffeine and is sweetened unnaturally, usually with white sugar, which gobbles up useful B vitamins in the body and tends to put on the pounds. Vegans like to eat carob instead of milk chocolate, which contains all the above things plus milk, a known dairy product. Carob flour is good to use as a substitute for chocolate powder when baking.

Here's a dairy-free dessert that uses carob flour, kuzu (root starch) and agar-agar (gelatin from the sea — see "kanten"): Put a heatproof bowl in some boiling water and add 2 cups of soy milk, 1 tbsp. of raisins, 1 tsp. carob flour, 1 tsp. kuzu (dissolved in a cup of water), and a pinch of cinnamon, and let get hot. Add 1 tbsp. barley malt and 1.5 tbsp. agar-agar and stir until creamy. Allow to cool a little, pour into a mold, let set, and serve with a fistful of fruit.

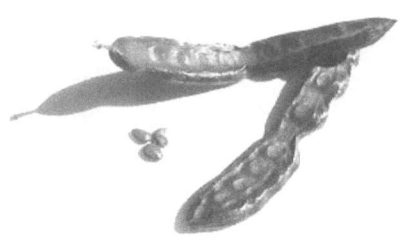

like it or lump it, is the second in a series of sea vegetables featured on my menu. This one is a red algae (it actually turns yellow or white after it is dried by the sun) that is also called Irish Moss due to its abundance in that land, where it is used to treat lung diseases and to help make the beer more clear. Because if its tendency to get gooey when added to certain liquids (like water) it is used commercially in other lands to emulsify or stabilize stuff like ice cream, fruit syrup, cheese, and instant soup, and to make other, non-food items like makeup and glue. In the humble home, it can be used to thicken soup, pudding, or to make a savory jelly, like so:

Soak a cup of carageen to make it soft, rinse it clean, then add it to 5 cups of boiling vegetable stock. Simmer for half an hour, then strain. This liquid makes a good base for thick soups. Irish Moss can also be fried or sautéed with vegetables.

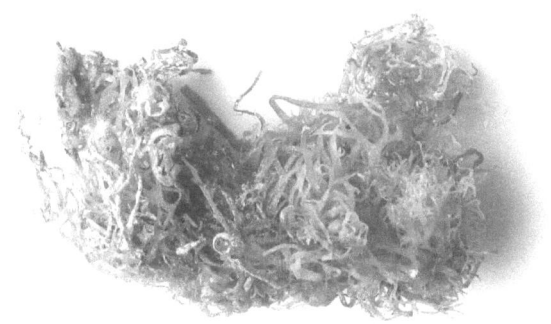

http://www.dkimages.com

The household name of this helpful herb, which grows as a woody vine in the rainforests of South America, comes from the small, hooked thorns at the base of its leaves that allow it to climb trees up to 100 feet. As the "sacred herb of the rainforest," it's been used since the age of the Incas to strengthen the immune system and treat ailments of the innards, such as tumors, ulcers, and the like. Modern doctors also prescribe "una de gato" to treat arthritis, diabetes, chronic fatigue, asthma, herpes, and PMS, as well as to reduce the side effects of chemotherapy. Last but not least, it's being used in conjunction with AZT to treat AIDS, and has been shown to raise T-cell counts much more than AZT alone. The healing ingredients in cat's claw are alkaloids with fancy names like rhynchophylline, pteropodine, and isopteropodine, plus tannins, which team up to increase circulation and immune response. Because of the demand for cat's claw, some indigenous groups in Peru are able to make a living by collecting the stuff from the jungle. The root and the bark of the vine are equally curative, but harvesting the root has been made illegal, as that tends to kill the plant and mess up the ecosystem. So, if you're buying cat's claw extract or capsules, make sure to get the kind that comes from the bark.

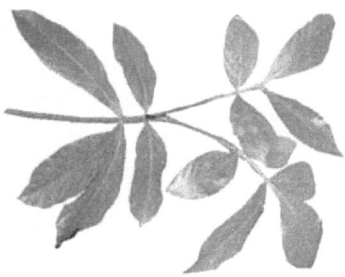

http://www.nutridirect.co.uk

CAYENNE

All pepper varieties hail from the Americas and share the genus *capsicum*, a word derived from the Greek word "kapto," which means "to bite." It's this hotness which led European explorers to call the fruits of these plants "peppers," after the coveted spice made from ground peppercorns (which come from an unrelated Asian plant). Cayenne peppers, which may have originated in west Africa, share their name with a river in French Guiana, which may have gotten its name from a Caribbean Indian word, "kian." At any rate, this long, tapered, red pepper contains lots of Vitamin C and iron, and has been used for ages as a metabolism booster and pain reliever. Its active ingredient, capsaicin, stimulates the digestive juices and increases blood flow, thereby strengthening the pulse, lowering blood pressure and maybe cholesterol levels, and fighting fatigue by moving oxygen to the muscles. As a pain reliever, capsaicin causes the release of a pain neurotransmitter called "Substance P," which eventually gets depleted from nerve cells (this is how it's possible to develop a tolerance for spicy foods). The usual effect of capsaicin as a pain reliever, though, is to divert attention from the original pain, as is the case with certain capsaicin-containing ointments like "Heet." The healthful effects of cayenne are said to increase with its spiciness, which in raw peppers is about 30,000 Scoville Units (comparable to Jalapeno, while the notorious habanero packs around 300,000 SUs). Cayenne powder, made from dried, ground peppers (not always or exclusively cayenne) has about 5,000 SUs. Although used mainly in cooking, it's also sold these days in tablets or caplets, often combined with other herbs because of its ability to help with their assimilation.

CELERIAC,

a.k.a. celery root or knob, is actually a member of the pars-ley family, which includes carrots, parsnips, and fennel. This lumpy, frumpy vegetable is fairly popular in northern Europe, but elsewhere hasn't gotten the attention and love it deserves. It's low in sodium and calories, high in fiber, vitamin C, calcium, and potassium, and has antioxidants that boost resistance to colds and flu. In the store, look for base-ball-sized tubers that feel firm and dense. After you cut off its stubby stalks, little rootlets, and brown peel, celeriac can be grated and eaten raw in salads, boiled in soup, or sliced and tossed in a tangy mustard remoulade like in France. It also goes well with potatoes, turnips, parsnips, or carrots, as in this simple recipe:

Bring 3/4 cup water, 1 tbsp. olive oil, 2 tbsp. lemon juice, 1 tbsp. natural sweetener, and 1/2 tsp salt to a boil. Add 3 diced carrots, simmer for a few minutes, then stir in one peeled, julienned celery root and simmer until the vegetables are soft.

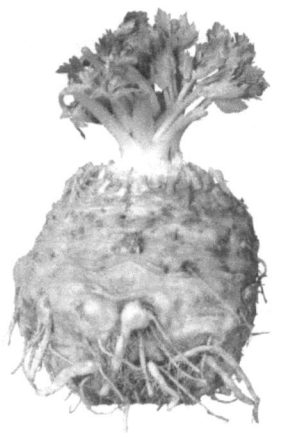

http://localfoodtastesbetter.files.wordpress.com

grow in twisty, hook-shaped pods and come in many colors, including white, yellow, red, brown, and blackish. They're called "garbanzo" beans in Spain, "ceci" in Italy, "pois chiche" in France, and "Bengal gram" in India, the world's main producer. They're also referred to as "Egyptian peas" because they used to grow wild over there back in pharoah days, though they probably originated somewhere else, like in Turkey. From there they were brought by traders and explorers to other lands like the Middle East, where they really caught on. People there roast them whole, grind them into flour, cook and mash them into *hummus*, or cook and mash and fry them into *falafel* (patties sometimes seen peeking out of pitas). These peas are high in calcium, phosphorus, iron, and protein. Like other legumes, when germinated, the sprouts provide lots of vitamins A, E, and B (maybe even B12, which is hard to get from plants), and more vitamin C than citrus fruit. Garbanzos need to be soaked for a long time, like overnight if possible, and take about 2 hours to cook. Use about 4 cups of water per cup of beans.

To make a basic hummus spread, blend 1-1/2 cups cooked beans, 2 or 3 cloves crushed garlic, a few tablespoons of tahini, and the juice of two lemons together to make a paste. If you prefer a creamier kind of dip, add a bit of olive oil or water to the mixture. You can also throw in a little tamari, salt, parsely, pepper, cumin or whatever tickles your fancy.

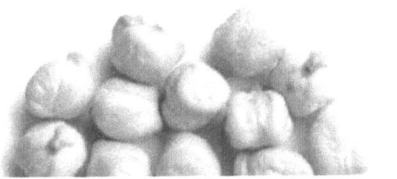

http://lifedirector.files.wordpress.com

CHILE PEPPERS

The word "chile" (as opposed to "chili," which usually refers to the dish made with beans) comes not from the skinny South American country, but from the pepper's place of origin in Central America, where the Aztec word "chil" referred to the spicy species growing in that region as early as 7,000 BCE. The word "pepper," meanwhile, was coined by none other than Chris Columbus, who tasted the stuff on his American vacation in 1493 and saw a cheap substitute for black pepper (*piper nigrum*), which was in big demand in Europe at the time. All 26 or so known species of pepper come from perennial shrubs related to tomato, potato, and eggplant, and share the genus *capsicum*, which means "to bite" in Greek, although some bite harder than others. The most vicous is probably the habanero, which registers about 300,000 Scoville Units, compared to jalapeno's 5,000 SUs, while sweet bells barely tip the scale. The fiery ingredient is called "capsaicin," which is concentrated mostly in the connective tissue or pith, and increases in quantity as a pepper ripens (usually from green to yellow to red). This oily chemical affects heat receptors in the brain, which put the body into cool-down mode, causing increased heart rate and metabolism, sweating, and a snotty nose. This "mucokinetic" reaction was noted early on by Hippocrates, who prescribed pepper and vinegar potions to cure respiratory ailments. Modern scientists, noting that people in Mexico have a fairly low rate of heart disease, think capsaicin may break down fat and clots in the blood. Capsaicin, by the way, is soluble in alcohol, not water, and is counteracted internally by dairy products and relieved externally by aloe vera. Frequent chile eaters will eventually build up a tolerance for the stuff. Apart from capsaicin and its possible health benefits, peppers contain more vitamin C than oranges, lots of vitamin A, plus calcium and potassium

CHLORELLA

Its name means "little green," and for good reason. This single-celled microalgae is about 100 times smaller, even, than spirulina, another itty-bitty "miracle food," but may be even more miraculous. It's been around for over 2 billion years, and was discovered in the late 1800s by a Dutch guy. The Germans studied it during WWII, and it's still the most-researched and most popular algae in the world. This "Jewel of the East" is about 60% protein, contains all the essential aminos and then some, and over 20 vitamins and minerals: plenty of vitamins C and E; more iron than, and 6 times as much vitamin A as, spinach; more of the elusive B12 than liver, and the highest concentration of chloropyll, nature's best detoxifier, in the whole wide plant world (20 times more than alfalfa and almost 10 times more than spirulina). It also has anti-cancer power and has been shown to reduce cholesterol and blood pressure. On top of it all, *chlorella pyrenoidosa* has huge levels of the nucleic acids RNA and DNA. Benjamin Frank, a studier of longevity, thinks that aging is caused by the loss of these chemicals. Their best source used to be canned sardines (a Floridian named Charlie Smith lived on them for the last 20 of his 137 year life), but, sorry Charlie, chlorella has many times more. A Dr. Fujimaki noticed that it grows darn fast (quadrupling in quantity in a day or so), and boiled out what he calls Chlorella Growth Factor (CGF). This regenerative energy booster was given to 10-year-olds, who grew almost twice as fast, and to mice, who lived 30% longer. Another great thing about chlorella: in 1 year, 1 acre can grow about 40 tons of it (that's over 20 tons of protein). The same acre would grow only 2 tons of rice and 1/2 ton of soybeans (but keep eating rice and beans, by all means.) Chlorella is available in powder or tablet form. It takes a few months after you start eating it for its effects to really kick in.

COLOSTRUM

After giving birth, mammalian mothers produce this nutritious substance for a few days before secreting breast milk. Although intended by Nature to help newborns grow quickly and fight off sickness, colostrum is being sold to adults as the latest, greatest way to stay (or get) healthy. In fact, if you believe Daniel Clark, who wrote a book on the stuff, colostrum is the "ultimate anti-aging, weight loss and immune supplement" if not the "perfect food." In addition to being packed with vitamins and minerals, it apparently contains two important kinds of chemicals: immunoglobulins and growth factors. The first group includes antibiotic, antiviral, and antibacterial chemicals like interluken, interferon, and protein-rich polypeptides (PRPs), all of which stimulate the lymphatic system; and lactoferrin, a protein that gets iron to red blood cells. The growth factors include insulin-like growth factor (IgF-1) and epidermal growth factor (EgF), substances that accelerate the healing of damaged tissue, repair DNA and RNA, burn fat and build muscle. Colostrum also contains glycoproteins that save all these helpful compounds from being broken down by stomach acids, friendly intestinal flora like acidophilus, bifidus, and lactobacillus, and chemicals that regulate blood sugar levels. Commercial colostrum, though taken from cows, supposedly contains the same nutrients as (and many times more immune factors than) human colostrum. Unfortunately, much of it is frozen for shipment (which affects its water-solubility), heat-processed (which renders it less active), or veterinary-grade (not harmful but not as beneficial), and none of it is FDA-approved (for whatever that's worth). Non-vegans may want to find capsules of colostrum from "organic" cows who have been fed grains and grass rather than hormones and other synthetic crud.

also called "mooli," is a long, radish-related root used frequently in Chinese cooking. It is said to be helpful in the breakdown of fat and mucous in the body, and to aid in the digestion of oily foods. Mooli makes a delicious side dish when grated and topped with tamari or vinegar, or it can be added to soups and stews like other veggies. Daikon greens, by the way, are also edible and quite nutritious.

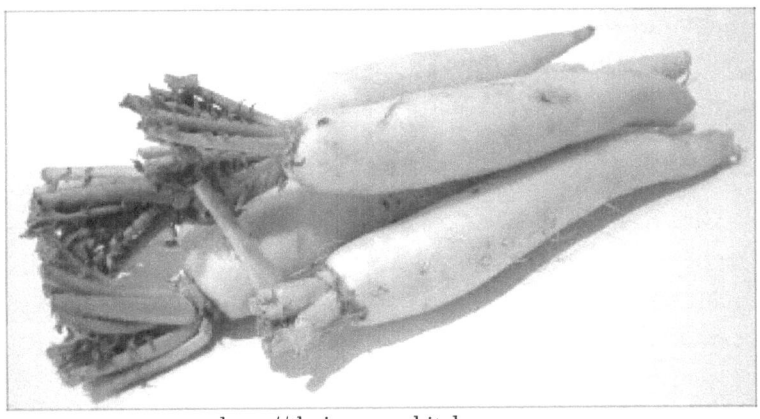

http://thejapanesekitchen.com

DAMIANA

Turnera aphrodisiaca is the botanical name for damiana, a small shrub native to Mexico and Central and South America, where it's harvested for its aromatic, medicinal leaves. The historical use of damiana dates back to the Ancient Mayans who ate the leaves to combat giddiness and loss of balance and to improve sexual function. Still an important component of folk medicine around the world, damiana's traits include antidepressant, diuretic, tonic, laxative, and sedative. Damiana has been purported to relieve headaches, treat coughs, control bed-wetting, promote menstrual discharge, and improve bladder function. Also, ingestion of damiana is said to produce a euphoria that lasts for 1 to 1 1/2 hours. Most popular, however, is damiana's association with treating sterility and impotence and increasing libido in both males and females. User be wary, however, for damiana may interfere with iron absorption and, when taken excessively for a long time, may cause damage to the liver. To prepare damiana tea, steep two heaping tablespoons of dried leaf in near boiling water for just under 5 minutes. Alternatively, one could prepare a liqueur by placing one ounce of damiana in one pint of vodka and letting the mixture sit for five days. Identified substances of damiana include volatile oil, gonzalitosin, arbutin, tannin, damianin, and beta-sitosterol. Though the chemical composition is not fully known, current studies have not isolated one chemical that would support its list of effects. In fact, some believe that the alcohol in damiana liqueur, rather than any chemical found in the leaves, is responsible for the aphrodisiac effects.

DONG QUAI

Alternatively called Dang Gui or Chinese Angelica, this tall-growing relative of celery can be recognized by its pale, green flowers, though it's actually prized for its root. As the most popular herb among women in China and the US, it's sometimes referred to as "female ginseng," used mostly to relieve menstrual cramps, PMS, and the hot flashes of menopause. Surprisingly, though, *Angelica senensis* works it magic not on the hormones but on the smooth muscles of the organs, so it's actually safe for guys, too. In fact, the herb has been used by both sexes at various times against anemia, arthritis, ulcers, insomnia, high cholesterol and blood pressure, and as a blood purifier and energy booster. Nutritionally, it's high in Vitamin A, B12, and iron, and extra-high in Vitamin E. The North American version of Dong Quai, *Angelica archangelica*, is called Angelica root, archangel root, or holy ghost root, and is traditionally put into a white, flannel bag or "mojo" to ward off evil or break a jinx. If ingested, the root has some of the effects of Chinese Angelica, though it's not as potent. Sold usually as a powder, sometimes in capsules or tea bags, Dong Quai should be avoided by pregnant women.

Dong quai root

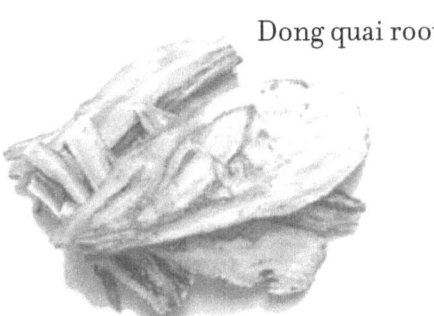

http://www.herbalremedypro.com

43

DULSE, WAKAME, HIJIKI

More sea vegetables! The composition of seawater is pretty similar to that of human blood, so its not surprising that underwater plants contain so many essential goodies.

After nori, **dulse** probably has the most appeal for western tummies. The lobed, wrinkled leaves of this algae come in a deep red color. Unlike most other sea veggies, dulse requires no pre-soaking and can be eaten right out of the bag, crumbled and sprinkled on soups and stews, or added to cooking beans to impart a subtle, smoky flavor. It's got lots of essential aminos and iodine, and is said to have a calming and balancing effect on the body.

Wakame is a brown algae (it turns deep green after soaking for 5-10 minutes) that's actually more popular than sushi nori. You've probably seen it floating in your miso soup, but it can be also tossed into salads or stir-fries.

Hijiki (or hiziki) is probably the most elegant sea vegetable. Its fine strands quadruple in size when hydrated, and have a distinctly briny taste. Hijiki has 20% more calcium than milk per serving, plus a goodly amount of iron, iodine, phosphorus and potassium.

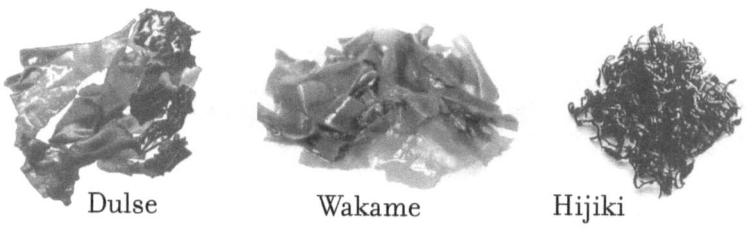

Dulse   Wakame   Hijiki

img.quamut.com//static.biotech-weblog.com//www.dkimages.com

DUNALIELLA

Among scientists, this one-celled microorganism is known as *Dunaliella salina* and classified as "halophilic," meaning that it thrives in very salty water, like that of the Dead Sea or the northern part of Utah's Great Salt Lake. It could also be described as "halotolerant," or capable of surviving in places as inhospitable as desert salt flats, to which it sometimes lends its green color (actually, the algae may turn red under certain conditions). At any rate, Dunaliella's claim to fame is that it's composed of up to 14% beta carotene, more than any other plant or algae. In fact, 3.5 ounces of dried Dunaliella is supposed to have as much beta carotene as 300 carrots. Beta carotene is also known as Provitamin A because it's easily converted by the liver into Vitamin A, a mighty antioxidant known to enhance the immune system and mental functioning, fight arthritis and prostate cancer, and help protect the skin from sunburn (when used with sunscreen vs. sunscreen by itself). Dunaliella also contains other free-radical-busting carotenes, as well as lutein and zeaxanthin, chemicals that help filter out certain harmful wavelengths of light that cause degeneration of the macula, part of the eye responsible for sharp and detailed vision. Dehydrated Dunaliella is usually sold as a supplement, often combined with other super-algae like spirulina and chlorella.

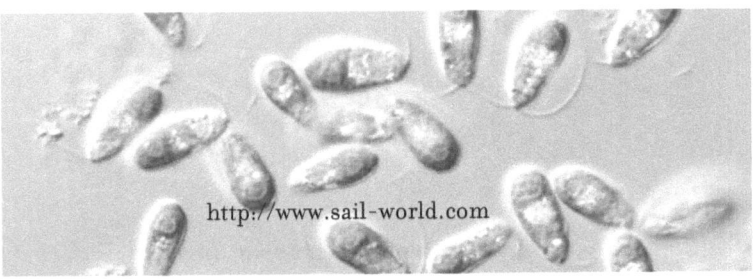

http://www.sail-world.com

EPAZOTE

(ehp-ah-ZOH-teh), *Chenopodium ambrosioides*, is a pungent, strong-flavored herb with both culinary and medicinal properties. This propitious plant has two aliases and may be found under the name of Mexican tea or wormseed. Indigenous to Mexico and South America, this perennial weed grows in the wild in many parts of the United States and Mexico, including roadsides and wastelands. In these parts of the country, however, epazote's flat, pointed leaves are usually found in the dried form. The flavor, which is so unique that it cannot be substituted by any other herb, is described as acidic, bitter, and lemony. Apparently an acquired taste, epazote can be added to beans, quesadillas, and the like to add flavor and to reduce the gas associated with bean consumption. Add two tablespoons to a pot of beans during the last thirty minutes of cooking to increase flavor and reduce gaseous side effects. In addition to this highly favorable carminative action, wormseed is also said to reduce pain and induce sweating, and its leaves and seeds are pressed into an oil for use as a vermifuge (known within the scientific community as "parasitic worm expeller"). Wormseed is particularly valuable as a vermifuge for children because of its efficacy, ease of administration, and low toxicity. Possible side effects of the concentrated oil form include allergic reaction and vertigo.

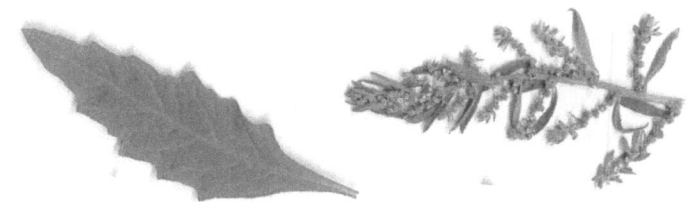

http://members.shaw.ca/bluemtnbio-dynamics

FAVA BEANS

These legumes are so ancient that nobody knows their original, wild source, but nowadays they're popular all over. In Italy, where the word "faba" means "bean," they're considered God's gift, while French folks have celebrations during the short, springtime growing season. They're eaten almost daily by the average Middle Easterner, and in China are seen fresh, dried, fried and salted, or sprouted. The English call them "broad" beans and used to call them "common" beans. They were brought to the New World in 1602, but never really became common in this neck of the woods, which is too bad because they're so good for you. They're low in calories (about 80 per cooked cup), high in protein, iron, potassium and fiber, with lots of A and C vitamins, and some of the Bs. Better yet, they contain lots of dopamine or L-dopa, a brain chemical that imparts energy, vitality and helps inter-noggin activities like memory retrieval. In fact, it's been shown that favas help people with Parkinson's disease. If picked and removed from their pods when young and small, favas can be eaten with their skins. With older, larger, ones, boil them for a minute, rinse them in cold water, then pinch the skins right off. They can then be fried with a little olive oil and thyme or sage, boiled and crushed with garlic, lemon juice, and olive oil, or boiled and tossed into a pasta or rice dish. Dried beans need to be soaked for 4 hours or more, then cooked for a little more than an hour. Favas are slightly bitter, kind of like my ex.

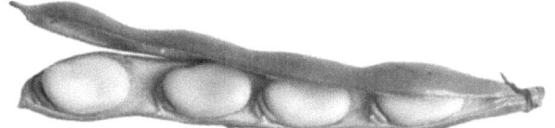

http://static-resources.goodguide.com

47

FENNEL

You can eat any old part of this easy-to-grow plant and reap some of its herbal goodness. Its leaves, best picked before the plant grows flowers, can be used in soups and salads or chopped up and added to vinegar-and-oil dressings to give flavor. The stalks can be boiled and eaten like a vegetable, and the seeds add a nice anise taste to baked goodies and to tea (the leaves are also good to steep). All parts, even the roots, have lots of iron, calcium, potassium, and the A and C vitamins. Foeniculum vulgae is not only good going down, but soothing to your tummy when it gets there. It stimulates the appetite, helps with digestion, and will relieve or prevent excessive flatulence (pardon my latin). It's sometimes used in cough syrup because it's good for coughs and bronchitis and because it tastes so lovely. It increases the flow of milk for nursing moms and relieves hot flashes for women in that particular phase of life. Oil made from fennel can even ease aching muscles and that pesky rheumatism.

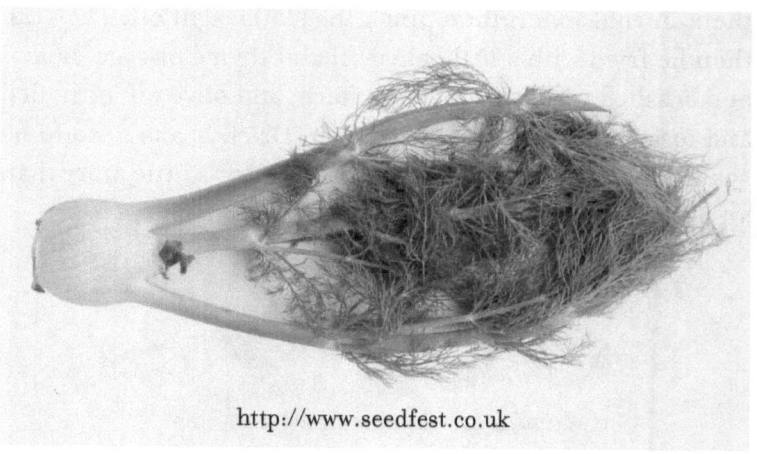

http://www.seedfest.co.uk

FIDDLEHEAD FERNS

For the two weeks before they unfurl, the leaves of this plant are coiled into a dark green spiral that looks kind of like the end of a violin. These edible coils were once a popular spring veggie with Native Americans and a little later with palefaced settlers. Today they're making more and more appearances in restaurants as a sort of delicacy, and can also be seen in Indonesian dishes. Also called "ostrich fern" or "pohole," fiddleheads are chewy, taste a little like asparagus or green beans, and are high in vitamins A and C. They can be eaten raw, although I'd recommend cooking them in one of the usual ways of steaming, simmering or sautéeing (you can then chill them if you want to go the salad route).

To make a simple and elegant soup, boil four or five fiddleheads until they're pale green and almost tender (about 7 minutes), then chop and set them aside. Sautée a minced onion until translucent, add 2 cups of vegetable stock, and boil the ferns until soft. Add 2 cups of soy milk and bring to a near-boil, then add 1/2 tsp. of lemon zest, and salt and pepper to taste.

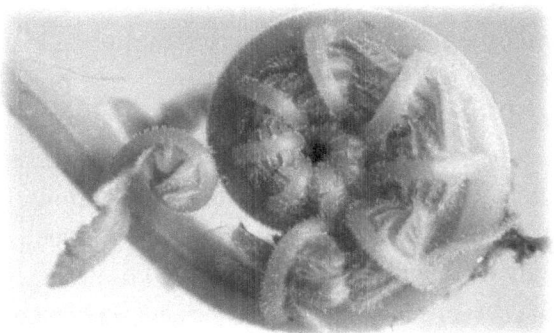

http://gallery.photo.net

FLAX SEED

Native to Europe and Asia, flax is one of the world's oldest cultivated plants. Linen, made with flax, was probably the first textile fiber used by humans. It's more durable than cotton, which is maybe why the Egyptians wrapped mummies with it. Anyhow, the roundish, brown seeds of this plant are the planet's best and healthiest source of essential fatty acids, containing 57% Alpha Linolenic Acid (twice the amount of fish oil) and a good amount of Linoleic Acid as well. So what's so essential about these fatty acids? Well, they're needed to build muscle and help tired muscles recover, they keep the hair and skin healthy and the blood flowing nicely, and prevent (or relieve) arthritis, high blood pressure, diabetes, and muscular dystrophy. The body can't produce these good fats on its own, and unfortunately, most people don't get enough of them (they're usually processed out of foods to extend shelf life), and get too many troublemaking saturated fats. I should say, though, that in order for EFAs to do their stuff, the body needs enough A, C, E, and B3 vitamins, and minerals like selenium, zinc and manganese. Besides EFAs, flax seeds contain lots of "lignans," plant chemicals that relieve menopausal symptoms and have antiviral and anticancer effects. Because of the high mucilage content of flax seeds, boling them results in a pasty mush, but they can be eaten raw, ground up, or pressed (preferably cold) to make flaxseed (a.k.a. linseed) oil. Raw seeds have the most lignans, but some doctors, including one who cured schizophrenia with flaxseed oil, recommend taking a teaspoon of it every day, preferably with borage seed oil, which contains lots of complementary Gamma Linoleic Acid.

To make a dressing, mix 1/4 cup flaxseed oil, 1/4 cup water, 3 tbsp. lemon juice, 2 tbsp. fresh basil, and 1 tsp. finely chopped garlic.

FO-TI

Known as "Ho Shu Wu" in China, this functional food comes from the roots of *Polygonum multiflorum*, a Japanese evergreen. In Asia, it's prized by older folks as an elixir capable of restoring youthfulness, fertility, vigor, and even hair color, while people of all ages use it to calm an upset stomach, purify the blood, lower high blood pressure and cholesterol, and give a general jolt to the immune system. Fo-ti also has anti-inflammatory effects that are due to chemicals called glycosides. Apparently the plant's older roots are the more prized, as are those of a certain shape. After being dried, they're usually ground and then sold either as unprocessed, white fo-ti, or combined with a liquid made from black beans and sold as red fo-ti.

Fo-ti root

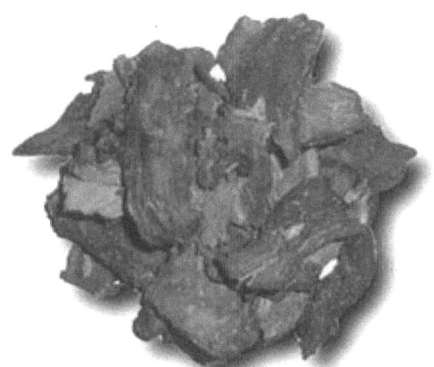

http://www.nutralegacy.com

51

GALANGAL ROOT

The tropical perennial from which this rhizome comes is a relative of ginger. Its name, in fact, was probably derived from the Arabic word "khalanjan," which may come from a Chinese word that refers to ginger. The root itself, dug when the plant is about 5 years old, is reddish brown outside and pale inside, with a flavor somewhere between ginger and pepper that's made it a popular spice in Southeast Asia, Iran, and even Europe, where it's also considered an aphrodesiac. In Russia, it's a flavoring for vinegar and liquor, while in India, its oil is used in perfumes. Galangal root's most popular medicinal use is to relieve motion sickness and upset stomach, but it's also been used against sore throat, infection, fever, and in some countries as a stimulant (sometimes in snuff) and even as a mild hallucinogen. Galangal, known in Malaysia as "lengkaus," actually comes in two varieties: Lesser galangal (*Alpinia officinarum*), which hails from Southern China, and the more common Greater galangal (*Maranta* or *Langka galanga*), which has its origins in Java, Indonesia. The latter species, with roots that are smaller and spicier, is especially popular in Thailand, where it's called "kha." There and elsewhere, the dried, powdered root (sometimes called "laos") is often combined with lemongrass to flavor soups and curries. Galangal root is also sold in dried chunks which need to be ground, or less commonly in its fresh form.

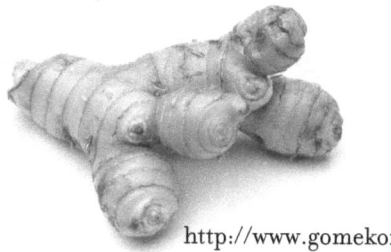

http://www.gomekongriver.com

52

GARLIC

is a member of the lily family and of the genus *Allium* ("odorous" in Latin), which includes onions, chives, and leeks. When the cells of these bulbous plants get ruptured or cut, they release sulfur compounds that react with the water in the eyes to form sulfuric acid, which makes those peepers leak even more. To avoid this tearful scene, slice underwater or wear swim goggles like my roommate. Anyway, the notorious "stinking rose" is native to Siberia, was brought to Egypt (archaelologists found some in King Tut's tomb), then to India and the Far East, and later to Europe. Over the centuries it has been used to ward off things like the common cold, tooth and head aches, arthritis, gray hair, obesity, insanity, vampires, or the "evil eye," and to improve things like eyesight, the voice, and sex drive. Studies performed in recent times indicate that some of them smelly sulfur chemicals (especially a couple called allicin and ajoene) may boost immunity, kill bacteria and perhaps even cancer cells, and lower cholesterol and high blood pressure. In addition to those off-putting but helpful compounds, garlic contains a good supply of vitamins A, B, and C, potassium, phosphorus, and selenium, which does help the immune system. If a garlic clove is planted to early, it will grow into one large bulb sometimes called a garlic onion, which will produce a normal cluster of cloves if planted. Elephant garlic, by the way, is actually a kind of leek.

http://vegetarianorganicblog.com

53

comes from the herby, tropical *Zinger officinale*, a member of the family of plants that also includes cardomom and turmeric. The part that people eat, the rhizome or root, is brown on the outside and pale or golden on the inside and is sometimes called a "hand" or "finger" because that's sort of what it looks like. It has a fresh fragrance and tangy taste, so it's often used as a spice or condiment, either grated, sliced, or pickled (sometimes served with sushi). In Southeast Asia, where ginger probably first grew, pieces are put into tea or directly into hot water to make a flavorful drink. Ginger can also be used to make a compress that will help stiff joints and muscles, stomach aches, constipation (or its opposite), kidney and sinus troubles, and toothaches. Here's how: Wrap about 3 tablespoons of freshly-grated ginger in a piece of cheesecloth and let it sit in about 8 cups of almost-boiling water for about 10 minutes, then take it out, squeezing out the juice. Roll up a cotton towel and dip all but the ends (which you'll need to hold on to to wring out the excess) into the ginger water, and apply it to the afflicted area, covering it with another, dry towel to keep the in the heat. Repeat after the compress has cooled. Ginger can be stored in the fridge, either wrapped in plastic or peeled and bottled in sherry, or in the freezer, as frozen ginger is great for grating.

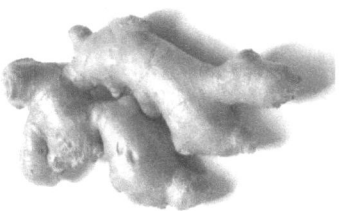

http://www.bonappetit.com

GINGKO

Forms of this hardy tree have been around for 200 million years, making it the oldest type on the planet. Individuals can grow to be 100 feet tall and 1000 years old, and seem to thrive even in smoggy cities. The Chinese have used the seeds and two-lobed leaves (which give it its species name, *biloba*) for ages to treat mental problems. The modern liquid or tablet form is the #1 most-prescribed herb in Europe (and getting there in the US) because of its role in improving brain functions and memory, especially in people with Alzheimers or Parkinson's. The stuff seems to open up blood vessels, increase production of ATP (the body's main energy chemical), and attack those "free radicals" that screw up brain activities. Gingko is also a good source of iron, vitamin C, and calcium.

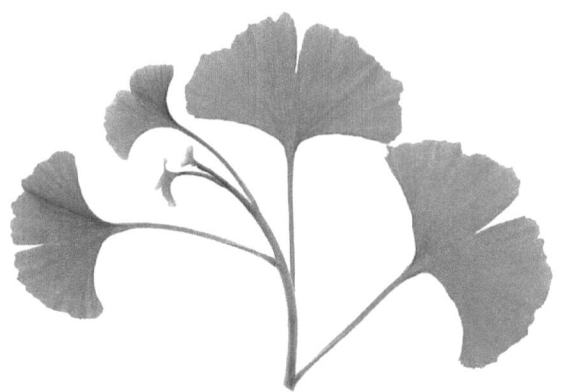

http://www.made-in-china.com

GINSENG

This famous medicinal root often grows in the shape of a person, so is sometimes called "man-root"(mostly by men, probably). It's also called the "Root of Heaven" because of its alleged power to increase strength, vitality, and lots of other things. In fact, the genus name, *panax*, means "all ills." It's been used in China for 5,000 years or more, and in North America for maybe just as long. During the Vietnam War, it was given to wounded soldiers to help them heal faster. There are a few different varieties: *Panax ginseng* comes from Asia (originally the mountains of Korea) and is has stimulating properties. Some of its magical ingredients are germanium, a blood purifier; saponins, which help metabolism; panasen, a brain chemical; and natural steroids for both boys and girls. It's sometimes put into soup. The north American type, *panax quinquefolium*, has more of a relaxing effect. It grows wild in some parts out east, and is cultivated in Ontario, where it used to be exported (mostly to Asia, by the way) almost as much as animal fur. Siberian ginseng, *eleutherococcus*, isn't technically ginseng at all, but has some of the same properties and antioxidants. All types of ginseng have a fair amount of minerals and B vitamins, are supposedly good for the glands, lungs, blood, and the immune system, and lower cholesterol while raising the old energy level with built-in "ginsenosides." Ginseng comes fresh, dried, powdered, in capsules, sodas, and teas, as an extract, or even as a spray for under the tongue.

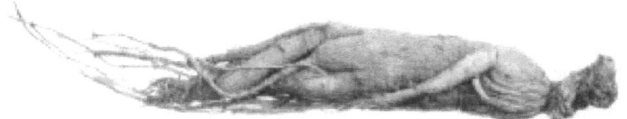

http://www.gnclivewell.com.au

GOJI BERRIES

Growing as a bush with vine-like branches, the perennial classified as *Lyceum barbarum* is often called "Chinese Wolfberry," revealing its country of origin. Although the shrub's leaves sometimes serve as raw material for salads, it's the bright red berries of "Gou Qi Zi" that are prized almost as highly as ginseng for their age-old role in strengthening vitality and curing disease. Word has it that residents of a certain region of Mongolia known as the West Elbow Plateau, who consume these berries daily (and, it should be noted, don't eat meat), share a life expectancy of well over 100 years and have no incidence of liver problems, arthritis, or other degenerative diseases. This anthropological discovery led Chinese researchers in the early '80s to conduct studies on the goji berry, which demonstrated its ability to lower high blood pressure, improve eyesight, inhibit cell mutation and tumor growth, and increase the production of white blood cells, thereby strengthening immunity. These medicinal benefits are mostly due to the stunning nutritional profile of goji berries, which consist of 13% protein by weight and contain more beta carotene than carrots, more vitamin C than oranges, 18 amino acids (including all 8 essentials), 21 essential minerals, and a goodly dose of Vitamins B_1, B_2, B_6, B_{12}, and E. Among the goji's other nutritional treasures are antioxidants called lycium polysaccharides, superoxide dismutase (SOD), and L-leucine, an essential amino acid not made by the body (but found in breast milk and other foods) that contributes to healthy muscle tone and increased immunity. With a sweet-tart taste similar to cranberries (or craisins), goji berries are finding their way into "power bars" and herbal teas, and can also be purchased in dried form.

(see front cover for image)

also called pennywort or centella, is an herb first used by Ayruvedic doctors in India to treat everything from schizophrenia to leprosy. It was also mentioned in a Chinese remedy book written about 2000 years ago. Nowadays, the leaves of this plant are eaten raw by folks in the Phillippes and by elephants in Sri Lanka and Africa, where most of it grows. Science has proven it to be good for circulation, so it's sometimes used to treat high blood pressure and vericose veins, and to speed healing. Its claim to fame, though, is that it seems to help people concentrate and stay alert. This might be partly because gotu kola boosts blood sugar levels, which, by the way, are often low in people with depression and mental illness. Unlike real "kola" plants, gota kola has no caffeine. It is, however, high in fiber, B vitamins, vitamin A, and minerals like aluminum and manganese.

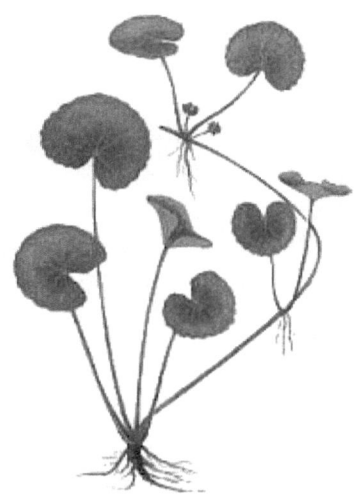

http://www.biotherapy-center.com

GRAPE SEEDS

So who are these "free radicals" we've heard so much about? They're actually unstable oxygen molecules that make metal rust, turn fresh apple slices to yukky brown, and cause damage and mutation in our cells, giving us cancer, degenerative diseases, and signs of premature aging. Unfortunately, they're everywhere, so you can't hide from their prescence, but you can eat foods containing lots of antioxidants. One the hottest antioxidants around is called Proanthocyanadin, said to be 20 times more powerful than vitamin C and 50 times more powerful than vitamin E in combating heart disease, cancer, Alzheimer's, arthritis, allergies, and protecting structural proteins like collagen and elastin that strengthen blood vessels, ligaments, and skin. This miracle chemical was "discovered" in the '50s by Jacques Masquelier, who also patented the name "Pycnogenol" to refer to Proanthocyanadin extracted specifically from pine tree bark. Later, Jacques found that the best place to get Proanthocyanadin is actually from the skins and seeds of regular, old grapes. The seeds of the purple variety, in fact, have a 95% concentration of this life-saver. All this may explain why the French, who drink wine with meals, can eat all that rich, fatty food and still have a fairly low rate of heart disease. In Healthy Helen's opinion, however, a little grapeseed extract beats a bottle of burgundy as a way to get antioxidized.

(see next page for image)

GRAPESEED OIL

is being touted by health-conscious folks as the oil of the future. It has half the fat of olive oil and is the only substance known that actually raises "good" cholesterol while lowering "bad" cholesterol. It also has one of the food world's highest concentrations (76%) of linoleic acid, an essential fatty acid that the body can't produce on its own (other good sources, you may remember, are flax seeds and hemp seeds). Its high vitamin E content contributes to its long shelf life, and its high flash point (the temperature at which it starts to smoke in the pan and break down into harmful compounds) makes it a good oil to sautée with. It can also be used cold in salads, where you may notice its subtle fruity taste. Fortunately, grape seeds are readily available as a by-product of winemaking, since white wine is fermented without the seeds. Most grapeseed oil, as you might expect, is imported from France and Italy. As with all oils, go for kind that's cold-pressed, since heat breaks down an oil's nutrients.

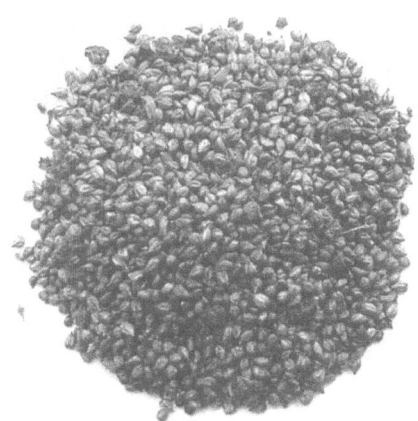

http://www.supplierlist.com

GREEN TEA

All three types of tea, whether black, Oolong, or green, come from the same plant; a hardy, tropical or subtropical evergreen bush called *camellia sinensis*, which first grew in China and was brought to Japan by Bhuddist monks who liked the buzz, and to India by British merchants who liked the bucks. Unlike green tea, black tea leaves are fermented (Oolong is semi-fermented), which ups the caffeine (black packs three times the punch of green). Of course, caffeine content is also affected by how long the tea steeps, as well as how big the leaves are (cutting and crushing make for easier extraction of the stimulant), and even their age when picked (younger=stronger). Fermentation also affects other chemicals called polyphenols, which get oxydized in the process, adding flavor and color and decreasing astringency. Unfermented and unoxydized green tea, then, has a subtler flavor and color, and is a bit bitter, but is better for you, containing more polyphenols, which aid digestion, boost immunity, and inhibit absorption of cholesterol. All teas, but especially green, contain cavity-fighting fluoride (green "gunpowder" tea has about 150 ppm, compared to about 1 measly ppm in fluoridated water). Green tea is also high in vitamin C, and, according to Dr. Fung-lung Chung (a real person), may also prevent lung disease and other cancers. Loose-leaf green tea requires about three minutes to steep (smaller leaves or bags infuse faster), and can usually be used a few times. It is not to be drunk with milk and sugar, unless you really want. To make iced tea, either make a double-strength batch and serve with ice, or put some normal-strength tea in the fridge until chilled. Green tea combined with roasted rice is called *genmaicha*, while *kukicha* is made from tea twigs and has even less caffeine than regular green.

GUARANA

Also called *Paullinia cupana*, Brazilian cocoa, uabono, or zoom, this South American perrennial grows as a vine in the wild and as a shrub in its domesticated form. The plant's small, reddish fruits contain dark seeds which have been used by Amazonian peoples for ages to treat malaria and dysentery, impart strength and crank up the old sex drive. The time-honored method of preparation involves collecting the seeds, dry roasting them, grinding them with a little water (and sometimes a bit of starchy cassava) to make a paste, and shaping the paste into brownish cylinders that are sun-dried and later grated into water to make a cocoa-like beverage. In ages past, "guaran sticks" were used as currency and were grated against the raspy tongue of a Piracuru fish. These days, they're a big thing with Brazilian miners, who drink guarana tea for energy. This energy comes mostly from the caffeine-like chemical guaranine, present at a concentration of about 5% (as opposed to coffee's 2% caffeine). This stimulant supposedly metabolizes more slowly than caffeine (perhaps because of guarana's fiber content), making for a longer-lasting buzz with fewer side effects. Guarana has been in use in Europe since 1817 (mostly as a headache remedy), and marketed in modern times as an appetite suppressant and anti-smoking product. It's been popular for many years as a soft drink ingredient in Brazil, and has more recently shown up in Pepsico's own "Josta." As the fourth largest harvest of the Brazilian rainforest, guarana fortunately grows quickly and doesn't take up much space, so it's considered sustainable. It's sold in sticks, as a powder, and in the syrup form used to make soda.

HEMP SEEDS

Cannabis sativa, which means something like "helpful hemp plant" in Latin, has been used for thousands of years to make everything from clothes to medicine to the Constitution of the US, where, nowadays, it'll help get you thrown in the pokey. The seeds of this versatile weed won't make you goofy, but they might make you healthy if you're not careful. In fact, they're being called "The Food of the New Millennium," beating out even the heavyweight champion of legumes, soybeans. Weighing in at 25% protein, hemp seeds are a little behind soy, but the proteins are easier to digest because they match up nicely with the ones already in the blood. The seeds have more iron, phosphorus, B vitamins, and way more fiber than soybeans, and hold their own in the A and E vitamins department. The real strength of these nutritional nuggets, though, is in their oil, which makes up 35% of their mass. A good 80% of that is unsaturated linoleic acid (LA) and linolenic acid (LNA), which supposedly exist in an ideal 3:1 ratio. In other words, hemp seeds have more essential fatty acids (in the most usable proportions) than any other edible thing. Essential fatty acids help get energy out of food and into the body, aid the immune system and the brain, add luster to the skin, hair, and eyeballs, and basically contribute to the body's growth and vitality, so they're pretty important. Most people don't get enough of them and get too much saturated fat, which make the friendly fats degenerate into unfriendly cancer-causers. It's against American law to grow hemp seeds, but it's okay to import them if they've been sterilized. They can then be roasted, ground into butter or flour, or thrown into salads, bakery, or just about anything. A handful will provide a grown-up with enough protein and EFAs for the whole day. Supposedly the Bhudda survived for awhile on just one hemp seed a day, and he turned out to be a pretty smart guy.

Known to botanists as *Ocimum sanctum*, this healthful herb is indigenous to India, where it can be found growing in flower pots and gardens in and around most homes. Since the ancient Vedic period, tulsi (or tulsee), as it's called, has been considered by Hindus to be an earthly form of the goddess Vrindivani, an associate of Vishnu the Preserver. Indeed, Ayurvedic practitioners classify the plant as *saatvic* or good for maintaining general well-being, and have used it to prevent specific ailments like colds, fever, and malaria, as well as to treat other problems of the digestive and respiratory systems. Western science labels Holy Basil an adaptogen, capable of counteracting the effects of stress on the body, and has found that it also seems to lower cholesterol and benefit people with cataracts. Its antibacterial and antifungal properties make the herb a popular ingredient in salves, balms, and even toothpaste, like the common Indian brand, "Dabur." Like its relative Sweet Basil, Holy Basil is used in cooking and salads, though traditionally it's simply boiled with honey to make a rejuvenating tea. Like most herbs, it's also sold in pills or as an extract.

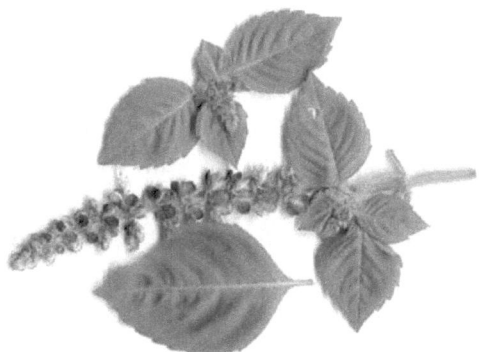

http://oldvegiepatch1972.googlepages.com

was one of the first foods that the native Americans gave to the white people that landed in their land way back when. It is made from the biggest part of the corn kernel, the part that scientists like to call the endosperm (tsk), which is not the hull (the outside part), nor the germ (the tiny, inside seed part). In the olden times, hominy was made by soaking dried kernels of corn (usually the white kind in the South and the yellow kind up North) in lye water for a couple days until the hulls came off, then cooking the stuff until puffy. Nowadays, hominy can be made in the home using baking soda instead of lye, or by steaming those hulls right off, like they do over at Manning's, where they make what was, in 1904, the first canned brand. Hominy is also sold dried, usually enriched with things like thiamine, niacin, and riboflavin. Hominy is often crushed (or cracked, as Jimmy's uncaring friend might sing) into particles called grits, which are cooked and served mainly as a side dish (though not just for breakfast) and also baked to make cornflakes. When ground up real fine, hominy becomes cornmeal. It is also used in making alcohol and wallpaper paste. Hominy itself is fat free, but the butter and milk sometimes used to prepare it is not. It can be made into patties and fried, or mixed with beans to make a stew or chili.

Try mixing a can with 1 cup quinoa (cooked in a couple cups of water), 2 cups of cooked beans (pinto, black, or kidney), 2 cups peeled tomatoes, and some spices like garlic, cumin, cilantro, pepper, or whatever your heart desires or your tummy requires.

JERUSALEM ARTICHOKE

This plant is not related to the artichoke, and it isn't from the Middle East. Somehow, the Italian word for sunflower, "girasole," got turned into "Jerusalem" over the years, and goodness knows how "artichoke" got in there. Anyway, *helianthus tuberosus* is a kind of sunflower from right here in North America. It was cultivated by Native Americans for its edible flowers and its tuber (the "artichoke" part), which looks like a knobby potato or a ginger root. A couple of the first white guys to eat this vegetable may have been Lewis and Clark. "Sunchokes," as they're often labeled in stores, are sometimes ground to make a sweet, nutty-flavored flour that's high in protein, calcium, phosphorus, potassium (about 2%), and especially iron. It's also prized as having the highest level of "fructooligosaccharides," carbohydrates that hang out in the bowels and make healthy "bifidobacteria" (or probacteria), which fight unhealthy bacteria like *e-coli* and others that cause high cholesterol, high blood pressure and intestinal problems. The tubers are hard to peel, so they're usually just boiled whole or cut into chunks, or eaten raw in salads.

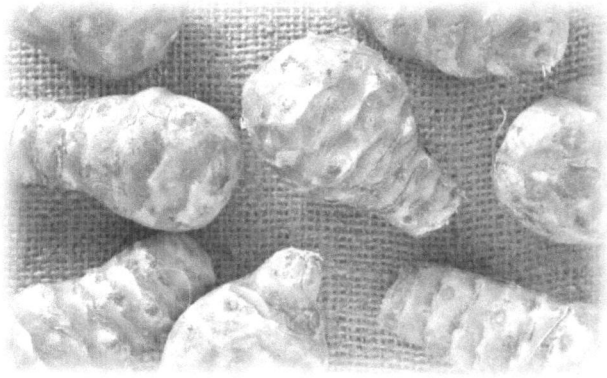

http://images.craveonline.com

JICAMA

(pronounced "hecama") is actually a Spanish word that refers to any edible root. In the US, however, jicama typically refers to a specific starchy tuber that also goes by the name yam bean, though it has no relation to the true yam. Regular folk might sometimes call it a Mexican turnip, while scientists have affectionately named it *Pachyrrhizus erosus*. Originally grown in Central America, the roots of this plant take 4-5 months to mature, at which time they contain about 10% starch and less than 1% protein. After peeling away the tough and rather ugly outside of this beet-shaped root, you will discover the juicy, crisp, white insides of the yam bean, which have been described as a cross between an apple and a waterchestnut. In fact, jicama can be used as a substitute for waterchestnuts in your favorite recipe. Eat it raw, boil it, or cook it, but don't try the leaves, stems, seeds, or ripe pods-they might be poisonous to humans.

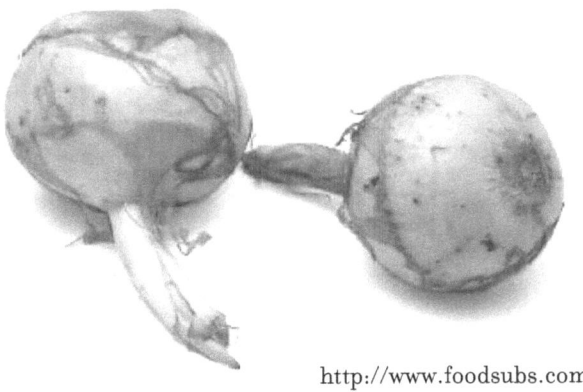

http://www.foodsubs.com

JOB'S TEARS

Coix lacryma-jobi is an ornamental grass that grows mostly in Asia and India whose name and claim to fame come from the tear-shaped beads that enclose its seed kernels. These hard, shiny, nuggets are about the size of cherry pits and range in color from off white to dark gray. They are usually used to make jewelery and rosaries, but a softer-shelled variety known as Hato Mugi Barley is eaten as a cereal. These grains, which resemble an oversized pearl barley with brown indentations in them, are higher in protein than brown rice and have lots of iron and calcium. On their own, they taste a bit grassy, but they make a chewy addition to soups and stews, and are especially tasty with (and nutritionally complemented by) split peas. They cook well when toasted first, then boiled in 2-1/2 cups water per cup grain. Being kind of starchy, they're best when freshly cooked, as they turn crunchy in the fridge and have to be rehydrated.

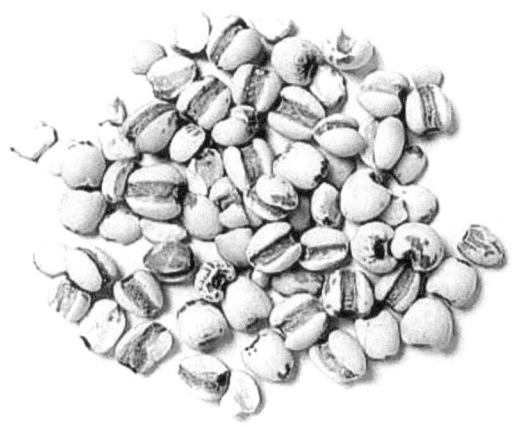

http://www.dkimages.com

KALE

is an old relative of the cabbage plant that hails from somewhere in the neighborhood of Asia Minor, but is now grown on cooler parts of the globe. In fact, modern types are pretty hardy and thrive in the fall and spring and are often eaten in the winter, which is why kale is called a "winter green." The edible leaves come in different shapes and colors, like bluish-green (Siberian) or grayish green (Scotch), but are generally thick, curly, frilly at the edges, and tend to get kind of rubbery when exposed to heat or left on a shelf. One variety called "Dinosaur kale" looks like a wierd, prehistoric palm tree. Kale is, of course, super nutritious, with only a little less vitamin A than carrots, more vitamin C per serving than orange juice, more calcium than milk, and plenty of iron for your blood and fiber for your guts. It's also got more protein than most other greens. Like other vegetables, kale can be used in salads, soups, stews, and stir frys. It's tasty when sautéed with olive oil and garlic or steamed and sprinkled with lemon juice.

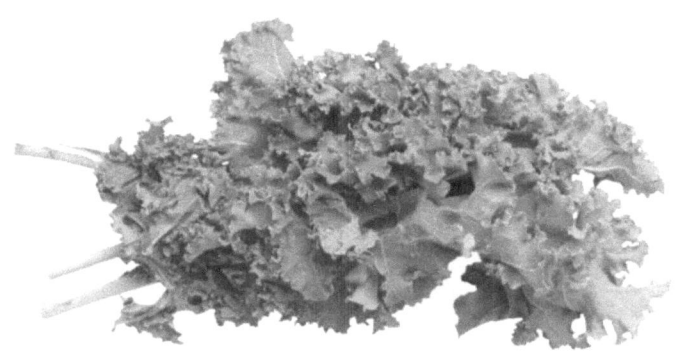

http://www.theallorganicfarm.com.au

KAMUT

(kah-moot) is a super-ancient ancestor of wheat. In 1949, a guy in the US Airforce aquired 3 dozen of its kernels, supposedly from an Egyptian pyramid, and mailed them to his dad in Montana, who planted them, then displayed the result at the fair as "King Tut's Wheat." In 1977, an agronomist named Bob Quinn, who was at that fair as a kid, found and analyzed some of the plump, golden kernels, which are about 3 times the size of regular (durham) berries. He named the plant "kamut" (Egyptian for "wheat"), but concluded that it probably originated in the Middle East. Anyway, along with having a wierd history, this food (which is still grown mostly in Montana), is delicious and nutritious to boot. Perhaps because it's not a hybrid like modern wheat, it has 30% more protein, more B and E vitamins, and is higher in 16 of 18 amino acids and 8 of 9 minerals, especially magnesium (23% more) and zinc (25% more). It's also safe for people who are sensitive to wheat, since it has almost no gluten (to make bread with kamut flour, mix with whole wheat flour). Many cooks consider kamut pasta to be of a superior texture. To cook "Egyptian wheat," use 1 part grain to 3 parts water, and simmer for 1-1/2 to 2 hours, until about 20% of the grains have burst open. They will be kind of chewy, with a rich buttery or nutty flavor. "Green kamut" is a powdered extract sold as a nutritionally outstanding superfood.

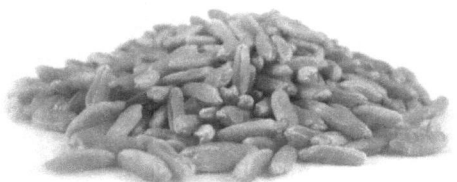

http://www.nutsonline.com

often called "agar-agar" in the west, is a gelatin-like substance made from red algae. The fronds are gathered by women divers in Japan, cleaned, boiled, allowed to harden, then cut into strips for drying and bleaching. This time-consuming process results in a flaky, brittle gelatin that melts in hot water (80°C or more) and, when cooled (under 35°C), sets more firmly than regular gelatin, which, incidentally, is made from discarded and boiled animal parts, like calves' hooves. Agar-agar is actually a different species of seaweed than the kanten described here, but it has pretty similar properties. It can be added to cooked, seasonal fruit and juice to make a jellied dessert.

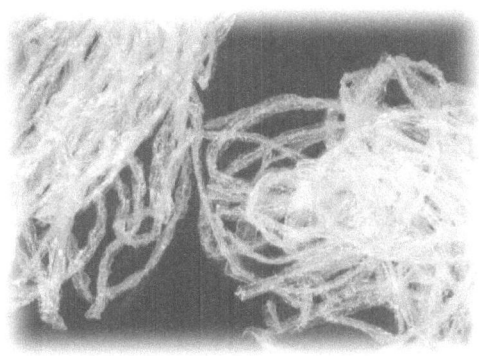

http://www.wingyipstore.co.uk

KAVA KAVA

This exotic-sounding herb, which grows mainly on an exotic-sounding, South Pacific island called Oceania, is a member of the pepper family. The first white fella to discover the plant, Captain James Cook, called it the "intoxicating pepper" because of its effect as a muscle relaxant and sedative. In ancient days, Polynesians used the roots of "sakan" to make a mildly narcotic beverage supposed to resolve conflicts at social gatherings. Kava kava first showed up in scientific literature around 1886, and today it's pretty popular in Europe (especially Germany) and is getting popular in the US as an anxiety-reducer and sleep improver. Most people prefer it to prescription drugs like Valium, probably because these benzodiazepines, which work on the brain, tend to cause mental impairment and lethargy, while kava kava works on the limbic or emotional system and can actually improve concentration and memory. An old-time herbalist named Brevoort once said of kava kava: "There is no other plant that gives such utter relaxation, while at the same time allowing such clear, penetrating mindfulness." The active chemicals in kava kava, concentrated mostly in the root, are lactones called (not surprisingly) kavalactones, which are absorbed quickly and go straight to the muscles to relieve tension. Over the years, kava kava has also been used against congestion and rheumatism, and as both an internal and external pain reliever. It is said to be safe and non-addictive, although it's not recommended for nursing moms or people with high blood pressure, doesn't mix wioth booze, and should, of course, be taken in moderation.

KIWIFRUIT

The climbing shrub that bears this fruit (which is actually a berry) comes from the Yangtse Valley in southern China, where "yang tso" has been used to make a restorative tonic since the time of the Khans in the 13th century. It wasn't until early this century that "Chinese Gooseberry" (*Actinidia chinensis*) was first exported as an ornamental plant, and not until 50 years after that that folks in New Zealand started cultivating its hairy berries and calling them "kiwifruit," probably after the flightless bird with a similarly fuzzy hide (New Zealanders, by the way, insist that the term "kiwis" applies either to the funny-looking birds or to citizens of New Zealand, not to fruit). Anyhow, around 2/3 of kiwifruit now comes from that sheep-filled island, the rest being grown in California, Africa, Europe – almost everywhere, in fact, but China. In a recent study conducted at Rutgers University, kiwifruit was ranked #1 among fruits in "nutritional density," based on the number of calories per 1% of the USRDA of a given nutrient. Ounce for ounce, it was found to contain twice as much Vitamin C as oranges (and 6 times as much as tomatoes), 75% more potassium than bananas, and more fiber than apples (as much as a whole grapefruit). It's surprisingly high in Vitamin E (which usually only comes in fatty foods like nuts, seeds, and oils) and apparently has goodly doses of calcium, magnesium, and Vitamin B6, as well as antioxidants like phenolics (found in red wine) and folic acid, a nutrient found in green veggies like broccoli and spinach that has been shown to reduce the chances of birth defects of the brain and nerves. Kiwifruit also contains "actinidin," an enzyme that breaks down proteins, which means it will tenderize your meat as well as melt through your jello. Although most people discard the suede-like skin (New Zealanders use it to repair bike tires and make pillowcases), it's perfectly edible and, in fact, nutritious. The bright green, seed-swirled flesh, meanwhile, tastes tangy and looks lovely. Try sliced kiwifruit as a substitute for tomatoes in a salad, or smashed kiwifruit as an alternative to applesauce.

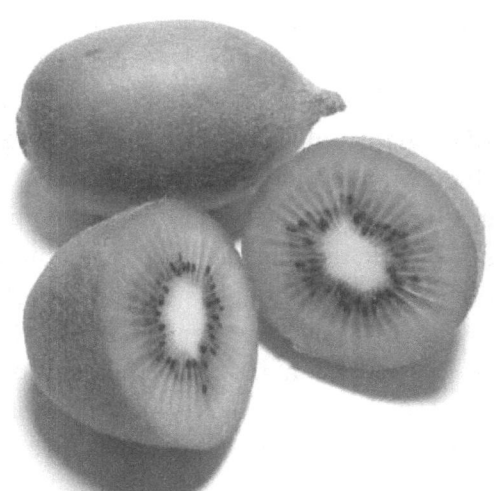

http://www1.sulekha.com

KOHLRABI

The first official reference to this vegetable was in the 1700s, but some say it's been grown for 2000 years or more. Nowadays, the "cabbage turnip" is popular in Eastern Europe, Asia, and Germany, where its common name comes from. It's actually the same species as broccoli, cauliflower, and brussel sprouts, each of which has been cultivated to emphasize certain traits of the plant. In kohlrabi's case, it's the bulbous, turnip-shaped stem base that gets the attention, although the spinchy leaves can also be eaten. The white, green, or purple stem, which rests on the ground as it grows, has a creamy-white interior that's high in vitamin C (a 1-cup serving gives 140% of the USRDA), potassium, calcium, and fiber. It can be steamed or boiled like most vegetables, or eaten raw in salads (it's especially yummy in the potato version).

To make a quick slaw, combine 6 peeled, shredded kohlrabis, 2 chopped apples, and 1 TB of sliced green onion with your favorite dressing.

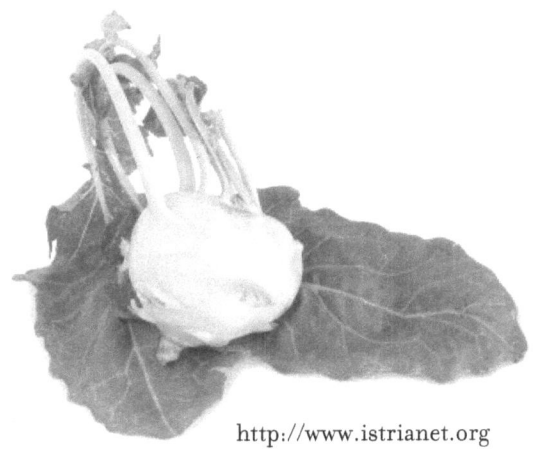

http://www.istrianet.org

KOMBU

is a type of brown algae (you're drooling already) that grows in deep water and whose fronds (the plant part) can grow up to 15 feet in length. This sea veggie contains an amino acid called glutamic acid, which mad scientists have successfully synthesized and sold as monosodium glutamate, an additive that, as Mrs. Dash knows, makes even the most bland food taste finger lickin' good. Kombu also contains plenty of iodine to help cure any goiters you might have. A strip of it can be added to a pot of beans to help them cook faster, give them a swift kick in the flavor department, and make them easier to digest (fewer flatulations/min). Its most popular use, however, is in the making of soup stock:

Add 1 piece (about 3" by 1 1/2") to 4-5 cups water and heat slowly, removing the kombu just before the water boils. It can be used a couple more times, or chopped and cooked with land-based vegetables.

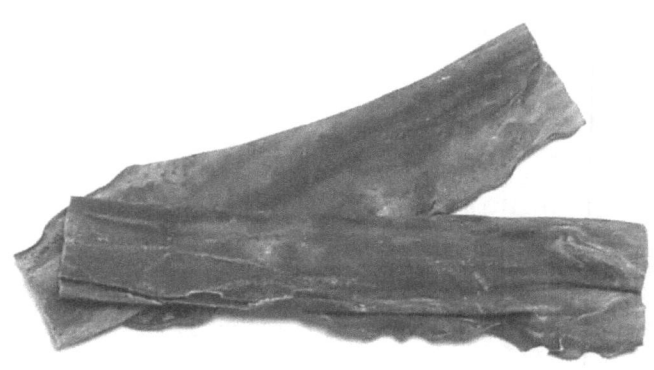

http://www.yale.edu

KOMBUCHA

Although a new thing in America, kombucha has supposedly been around since the Qin Dynasty (circa 250 BCE) in China, where the drink is called "Immortal Health Elixir." Its use eventually spread west to Russia and east to Japan, where it apparently got its name from a doctor named "Kombu" who served his tea or "cha" to the emperor. Confusingly, in Japan kombucha goes by the name *kocha kinoko* ("tea mushroom"), while kombu refers to a type of kelp (see previous page) that can also be used to make a tea. Outside of Japan, however, kombucha refers to a fermented drink made by a mass of microorganisms known as a "kombucha colony," or SCOBY ("Symbiotic Colony of Bacteria and Yeast") – not a mushroom. Kombucha is made by brewing a large batch of black tea sweetened with white sugar, letting it cool to room temperature, and then adding one of these rubbery pancakes to the mix. In a week to ten days, the colony will convert the tea's sugar and caffeine into B vitamins, minerals, antibiotic substances, lactic acid, amino acids, and glucuronic acid, which is thought to improve liver function. The resulting beverage is then strained and put into the fridge, which stops the fermentation process. Meanwhile, the SCOBY can be used immediately to ferment another batch of tea or produce another of its kind, sometimes called a "kombucha baby." While every batch varies in taste and fizziness, kombucha generally has a slightly acidic or vinegary taste and contains a trace amount of alcohol (about .5%). In the US, it is often touted as a probiotic used to increase friendly intestinal flora and thus improve digestion. Other reported health benefits include boosting the immune system, preventing cancer and curing hangovers. Despite its amazing qualities, kombucha is contraindicated for folks with candida problems, and certain batches may become contaminated with harmful microorganisms.

KUZU

Although native to the mountains of Japan, "kudzu" now grows like crazy in the southern US, wrapping its vines around trees and phone poles and covering anything in its path. The plant's roots, which can be yards long and as thick as your body, are usually ground into chalky chunks that are used as a thickening agent. These irregular, white bits dissolve quickly in cold water. If heated, the milky solution becomes clear and can then be added to soups, sauces, and jellies. Kuzu has been used to treat colds and digestive problems.

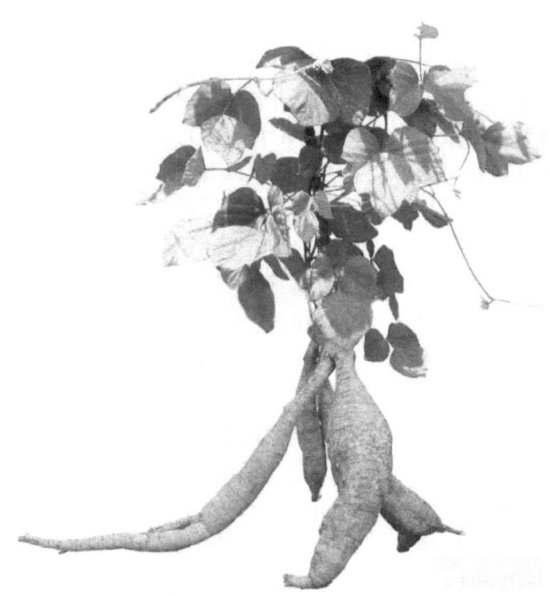

http://img.21food.com

LENTILS

are legumes that come, two per pod, from the annual *lens esculenta* plant that, in turn, comes from the near East. In the Bible, Jacob fixed his brother Esau a "mess of pottage" (or was it a "pot of message"?) that was made with lentils. Apparently they were brought to America by a Seventh Day Adventist from Germany who handed some to a fortunate farmer who started cultivating them. These beans have more protein than all others except soybeans, and are a good source of iron, phosphorus, and vitamin B, too. They come in a rainbow of colors, like black, brown, green, orange, yellow, red, and pink. Those last two types have the most protein, and are grown in India, where folks use them to make a delicious dish called dahl. In that part of the world, lentils are sometimes called "poor man's meat," but a person from America who might not eat meat and might also be a woman might want to just call them "lentils." Lentils don't need a lot of soaking–an hour or two should do. They also cook quicker than other beans, like in about 45 minutes. Use about four cups of water per cup of beans. When they get soft, add a little tamari or a pinch of salt and simmer another 20 minutes or so.

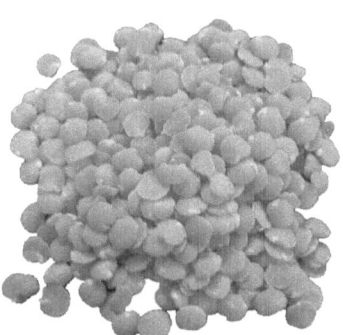

http://www.formaggiokitchen.com

79

comes from *Glycyrrhiza glabra*, a plant that grows wild in southern Europe and parts of Asia. It was found in King Tut's tomb, fed to the Roman legion, and has been a favorite of the Chinese since way back. It's still one of the most popular herbs in the world, used to purify the blood and lower cholesterol, fight fatigue and depression, stimulate the appetite for you-know-what, detoxify the liver and kidneys, and relieve arthritis, inflammation, bronchitis and sore throats. One of its ingredients, glycyrrhizin, is used in Japan to treat hepatitis and herpes, and may help fight cancer and HIV. Another substance, glycyrrhetinic acid, is used to treat ulcers, and a chemical called Inositol is necessary for brain cell activities. Licorice root also contains Vitamin E and some of the Bs, and minerals like phosphorus, manganese, and iodine. To top it all off, licorice root can be used a sweetener. Called "gan cao" ("sweet weed") in China, it is said to be fifty times sweeter than sugar cane. Unlike sugar, though, it's safe for diabetics and hypoglycemics (it seems to stabilize blood sugar levels), it supposedly quenches instead of increases thirst, and actually inhibits tooth decay. This root, though, is almost never used in candy (the flavor most people think of as "licorice" is actually an artificial anise flavor). Despite all of its goodness, licorice root may not be safe for folks who have high blood pressure or are pregnant.

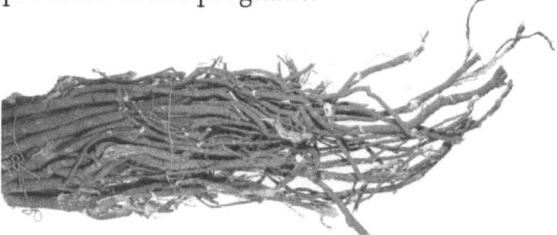

http://www.naturesflavors.com

LOTUS ROOT

The white lotus is the flower of summer in Chinese mythology, and a symbol of perfection, purity, and spiritual development in India. The less-sacred tuber of the plant grows horizontally in the mud of shallow ponds and somehow retains little air pockets, so that slicing results in an interesting and decorative cross-section. The off-white root can be eaten in salads or stir fries, or, like potatoes, boiled or even baked into exotic and holy chips (holy like swiss cheese, not the pope). It is high in vitamin C and iron and is said to relieve colds and congestion of the sinuses and lungs.

To make a tea, squeeze the juice from some fresh, grated lotus root into boiling water, add a little ginger and a pinch of sea salt, and simmer for a couple minutes. You can also buy the root dried in Asian food stores.

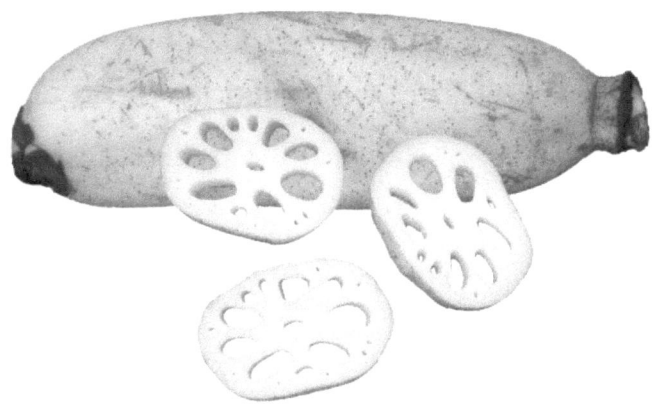

http://www.dpi.nsw.gov.au

LUPINS

The lupin plant was probably first cultivated by the Egyptians, but it now grows (in cruddy soil even) in Europe, Asia, Australia, and the Americas. Its flattish, whitish, beans are naturally bitter, containing alkaloids, which in some wilder varieties can be mildly toxic. Fortunately, a sweet lupin was developed in the US, but, unfortunately, it mostly gets fed to livestock. Humans, though, have been enjoying lupins (or lupini) for ages. Pliny, an old Roman, wrote: "No kind of fodder is more wholesome and light of digestion than the White Lupine. It will contribute a fresh colour and a cheerful countenance." The old-time herbalist Nick Culpepper noted that they're "good to destroy worms. Outwardly they are used against deformities of the skin, scabby ulcers, scald heads, and other cutaneous distempers," and John Parkinson backs him up by saying that many people "doe use the meale of Lupines mingled with the gall of a goate and some juyce of Lemons to make into a forme of a soft ointment," adding that burning lupins will drive away gnats. Modern scientists now know that lupins, at 30% protein, rival soybeans, and that they have even more calcium, are easier to digest, and have lots of iron as well. They are often made into gluten-free pasta called lupini, which supposedly never sticks to itself.

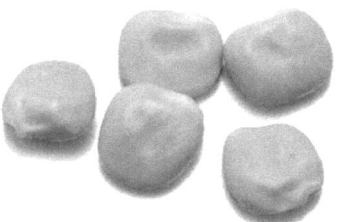

http://www.angryalmond.com

MACA

Like brussels sprouts, cauliflower, and cabbage, this perennial is considered a cruciferous plant; the only one, in fact, that's native to Peru. It also has the distinction of being the highest-altitude cultivated plant, flourishing at up to 15,000 feet in the rocky and barren highlands of the Andes. In these regions, its off-white, radish-like tuber has been a staple food and medicine for a couple millennia, although a botanical ancestor of *Lepidium meyenii* may have been used as much as 3,500 years ago by Incan warriors. The Spaniards who later exploited the land and its population were impressed by maca's ability to increase energy, stamina, and the fertility of their horses (and perhaps themselves), which led to increased demand and decreased supply of the once-abundant plant. These days, most so-called "Peruvian ginseng" (no relation to real, Asian ginseng) is of the species *L. peruvianum*, which nevertheless packs plenty of protein (10%), vitamins (B1, B2, B12, C and E) and minerals like calcium, magnesium, phosphorus, and especially iron and iodine. More and more doctors and naturopaths are prescribing maca to correct female hormonal imbalance and male impotence, improve mental clarity, combat chronic fatigue syndrome, and help with weight management. In general, it's considered an "adaptogen" capable of warding off the effects of stress on the body, as well as a "nervine" which nourishes and calms the nerves. Described as having a tangy taste and a smell like butterscotch, maca is traditionally baked like a potato (to which it is related) or stored (for up to 7 years without unsavory effects) and then boiled in water or milk to make a mushy porridge. Outside of Peru, maca is usually found in dried, powdered, and encapsulated form.

This herb, which comes from a weird-looking, nearly leaf-less shrub, was among the first to be listed by Shen-Nong, the Divine Ploughman Emperor, in an herb book he wrote a few thousand years BCE. Also called "ephedra" (the plant's genus name), its main use has been to treat respiratory problems like colds, flu, asthma, and hay fever. Native Americans, who used a different, indigenous species to make a drink, gave some to settlers in Utah in 1847, which led folks to call the herb "Mormon tea." Another of its names, "whorehouse tea," comes from the days when such a beverage was served in brothels because of the belief that it cured syphlis and gonorrhea, which it does not. What ephedra does do is open the bronchial passages and increase metabolism and heart rate. It also increases thermogenesis, or fat-burning, and is therefore sometimes sold as a weight loss product. It may also curb a person's hankering to smoke. The herb's active ingredients, in order of intensity, are ephedrine (most abundant in Chinese ephedra), psuedoephedrine (added to in Sudafed and other cold formulas), and norpsuedoephedrine (present in American ephedra). Most convenience stores sell synthetic ephedrine, often combined with caffeine, which enhances its effects, sometimes leading to nervousness, insmomnia, or even heart palpitations. It's this "speediness" which has led some states to outlaw ephedra, and the US Olympic Committee to include it as a banned substance. The FDA, meanwhile, considers it a drug of "undefined safety" because of its tendency to raise blood pressure. Interestingly, ma huang in its natural state has been shown to actually ease hypertension, and causes few unpleasant side effects when taken in moderation. Nevertheless, it is not recommended for people who are

MAITAKE

Pronounced "my-tah-kay," this mushroom variety is known in Japan as the "dancing mushroom," either because its overlapping, fan-shaped fruits look like dancing butterflies, or because a person who discovers these fruits might well jig with joy. The latter scenario was more likely back in Japan's feudal days, when the fungus was worth its weight in silver. These days, *Grifola frondosa* can also be found growing wild in Europe and the northern U.S (where it's called "Hen of the Woods" because its resemblance to fluffed-up chicken feathers), and has been artificially cultivated since the 80s. Like reishi and shitake, this super 'shroom is being hailed for its magical healing properties and handsome nutritional profile. While being incredibly low in calories, maitake is high in protein, fiber, iron, potassium, phosphorus, and vitamins A, B1, B2, B3, and biotin. It also contains a polysaccharide (sugar chain) called "D-fraction beta-glucan," which helps stabilize blood sugar levels, lower cholesterol and high blood pressure (up to 20% in a month in one study), and strengthen the immune system, including increasing T-cell activity in HIV and AIDS patients. Furthermore, maitake seems to slow the growth of cancerous tumors, and may reduce the effects of allergies and chronic fatigue. In Asia, maitake is usually sold in dried strips and used in soups and teas, while in America, it's most often found powdered and encapsulated.

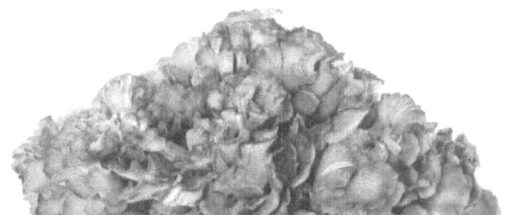

http://www.mushroomharvest.com

MANGOSTEEN

Completely unrelated to the mango, the mangosteen is a purple-red, apple-sized fruit that comes from the Purple Mangosteen tree, *Garcinia mangostana*, which grows in the tropics of Southeast Asia. In those parts, mangosteen rind has long been used to make a curative tea and a topical ointment. As legend has it, Queen Victoria once offered knighthood to anybody who could bring her a ripe mangosteen (nobody could), thus giving rise to its nickname, the "queen of fruits." Nowadays, mangosteen is being celebrated as a "superfruit," although the nutritional value is concentrated in the thick, reddish rind. Here one finds a bunch of chemicals called "xanthones" that may have anti-inflammatory, antimicrobial, antifungal, antiseptic and even anti-cancer effects. Meanwhile, the whitish, inner flesh lacks function but not deliciousness, with a sweet-tangy flavor resembling that of a peach. Until recently, mangosteen was not allowed into the US due to concerns about insects, but now it's available irradiated and imported from Thailand. One can also buy mangosteen juice. One popular brand, "Xango," is advertised as a "functional beverage," supposedly because it is made from the whole fruit.

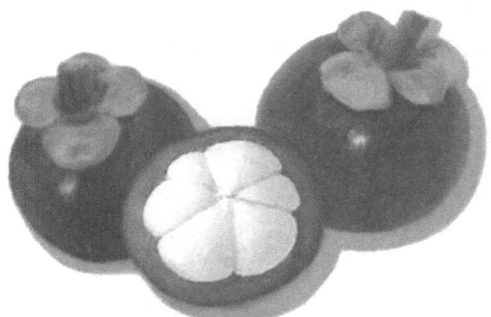

http://thaifruit.org

Named for its tendency to grow in areas wet and warm (it's also called "seashore mallow"), this tall, leafy perennial hails from the same family as hibiscus and okra, *Malvaceae*. Its consumption dates back to ancient Egypt, where the sap from its long roots was mixed with honey and taken to relieve coughs and sore throats. Ancient Syrians and Romans ate the herb as a veggie, as did the Greeks, who considered it a treatment for respiratory and digestive ailments, chapped skin, and wounds. In fact, it was the Greeks who contributed the word *altho* (meaning "to cure or heal") to the marsh mallow's botanical name, *Altheae officinalis*, while a specific Greek, Pliny, said, "Whosoever shall take a spoonful of the mallows shall that day be free of all diseases." In the 19th century, the term "marshmallow" came to refer to a concoction made by Europeans (who copied the Egyptians) from sugar, egg whites, and mallow sap that was given to kids with sore throats. What we now know as "marshmallows" are basically blobs of sugar, flour, and gelatin (which, by the way, also comes from ancient Egypt), and no longer have any connection to the plant, whose healing action comes from large carbohydrate molecules called mucilage. Marsh mallow, however, is still used medicinally (often combined with herbs like fenugreek), and is eaten in salads in France, where it's believed to be good for the kidneys.

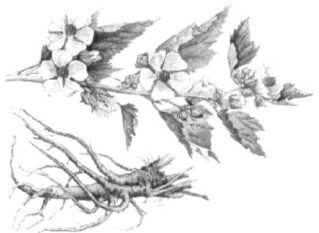

http://www.jmgkids.us

87

is a small, round, yellowish, gluten-less grain. It was once quite popular in China (before the introduction of rice) and Europe (during the seventeenth and eighteenth centuries it was more widely grown than wheat), and is still a staple in India, Korea, northern China, and many African countries. It is also the principal grain of the notoriously hearty Hunzas of the Himalayas. Elsewhere it is often sold unhulled and fed to birdies. Because of its alkaline qualities, millet is eaten by humans to cure acid indigestion and disorders of the spleen and pancreas. It contains gobs of protein, more iron than any other grain, and provides a good balance of amino acids. To cook this long-lasting and versatile food, add one cup (and a sprinkle of salt or soy) to about 4 cups of water, boil vigorously for 5 minutes, then cover and simmer, without stirring, for a half hour or so. Eat millet alone (by itself, not yourself) as a cereal or add vegetables to make a colorful dish.

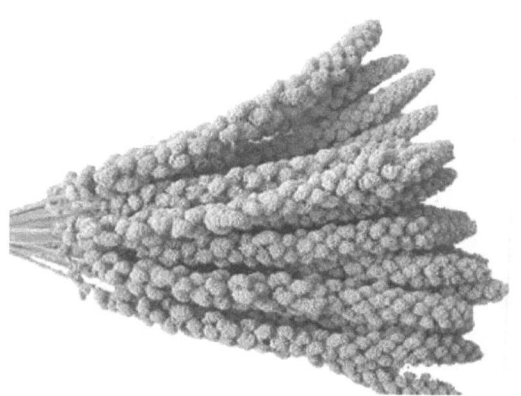

http://www.global-b2b-network.com

MISO

This traditional Japanese foodstuff is made with soybeans, salt, and a type of mold, *aspergillus oryze* (a.k.a. "koji"). Miso's consistency is generally pasty, but its color and flavor varies depending on the kind of grain used to cultivate the koji. For example, the thick, dark "hatcho" miso, known as the "food of the Samurai," is made with soybean koji and takes a few years to ferment, while "kome" miso, made with white rice, is sweet, light-colored, and ready in a few weeks. Other types include "mugi" (or country style) miso, made with barley, "soba" miso, made with buckwheat, "genmai" miso, made with brown rice, and "natto" miso, made with soybeans and ginger. All varieties contain complete proteins, B vitamins (including B12), antioxidants like vitamin E, essential fatty acids to lower cholesterol and isoflavones to fight cancer. Miso is usually diluted to flavor sauces and dressings, and to make the popular soup that accompanies most Japanese meals.

To make a fairly quick version, sautée a sliced onion with a few slices of ginger root, then toss in a couple sliced carrots and celery stalks. Add 4 or 5 cups of water, bring to a boil, and add about 4 tbs. of your favorite miso that's been diluted with vegetable broth or water. You can then add some tofu cubes, and maybe a drop of toasted sesame oil, and garnish with scallions or lemongrass.

MOCHI

is a traditional Japanese foodstuff made not from soybeans (believe it or not), but from glutinous (sticky) rice. The old-fashioned method involved steaming the unhulled (brown) grain in cedar boxes, then pounding and cutting it into flat cakes which were often enjoyed on festive occasions. White rice mochi was originally made only for princesses, who apparently were too busy to be bothered by nutrition. Believed to be a gift from the heavens, mochi is said to increase stamina and vigor as well as help bad blood and weak intestines. Ever so versatile, mochi can be toasted, fried, or baked (it puffs up like bread), eaten plain (it's naturally sweet and chewy) or with any number of other goodies. Spread it with hummus or peanut butter, stuff it with sautéed veggies or burrito fixings, or dip it in a mixture of soy, grated ginger, and honey.

To make a crispy dessert, spread 6 or 7 thinly-sliced apples on the bottom of a baking dish and top with 1/2 cup almonds or walnuts and 9 ounces of grated mochi. Bake at 350° for about 20 minutes, covered, then uncovered for another half hour or so until the mochi gets crunchy.

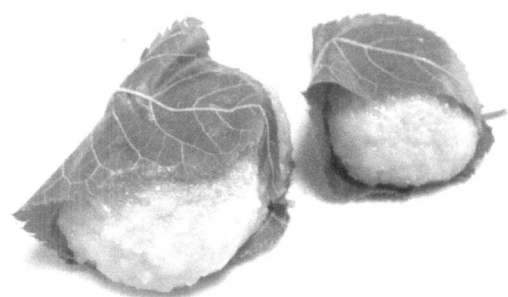

http://image.blog.livedoor.jp

is basically a by-product of the making of sugar from cane. The cane stalk is cut into chunks, smushed into a pulp, and the cane juice is concentrated and filtered to produce a sticky mixture called "massecuite." This goo is then spun in a centrifuge a few times to separate out the sugar (brown sugar still has a little molasses stuck to it). The last extraction yields "blackstrap" molasses, said to be the richest in nutrients of all sweeteners, containing more calcium than milk, more iron than eggs, lots of vitamin E and B vitamins, copper, magnesium, zinc, phosphorus, and more potassium than you can shake a stick of cane at. In fact, some people take a tablespoon, dissolved in a cup of water or spread on toast, as a natural supplement to help out with things like varicose veins, arthritis, ulcers, dermatitis, constipation, and nervous conditions. Unfortunately, though, along with all the goodies, blackstrap (and other types of molasses) may also contain lead, sulphur and pesticides used in the growing and processing. Your best bet, then, for a natural sweetener or sugar substitute is probably barley malt, a syrup made from plain old cooked barley. Unlike white sugar, it and molasses provide a slow and steady supply of energy for your busy body.

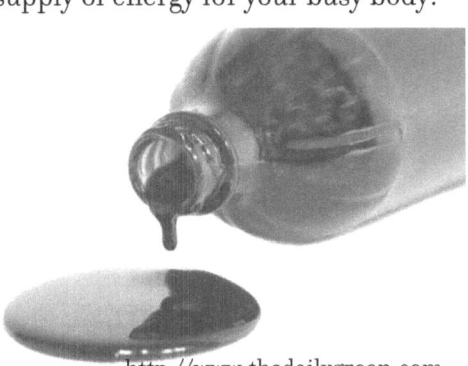

http://www.thedailygreen.com

MUNG BEANS

Whether called bundo, mongo, green gram, mash beans, or oorud beans, the fact is that about 98% of them are grown in Asia, as they have been for ages, although most come from a newfangled, disease-resistant variety of plant. It grows 1 to 2 feet tall and produces a dark, fuzzy pod full of small seeds that turn brown but are usually harvested when still green. These little legumes are usually germinated into crispy sprouts that are high in protein, vitamins A, B complex, C, and E, and minerals like calcium, potassium, magnesium, and phosphorus, but they can also be cooked up fairly quickly, without presoaking. In the Philippines, *ginisang munggo*, or sautéed mung beans, is a favorite dish, and folks there even toss the leaves of the plant into stews and stuff. Mung beans are also dried and ground into a flour that makes what Americans call cellophane noodles and Asians call harusame or saifun, which need only a few minutes of boiling, and are safe for people allergic to gluten.

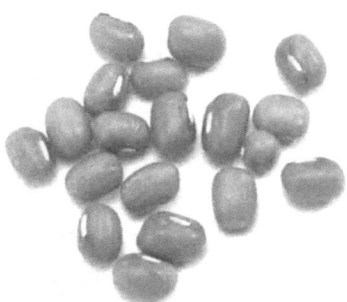

http://www.recipes4us.co.uk

NATTO

The name of this Japanese soyfood may come from "nassho," the word applied to the kitchen of a Buddhist temple, wherein such vegetarian fare might be concocted. The olden method involves covering a bunch of steamed soybeans with rice straw containing a natural bacteria called *natto bacillus*, then letting the beans ferment for a few days next to (or under) an open fire. This recipe dates back to at least 1000 years ago, when natto was popular enough to be peddled door-to-door in the old capital city of Edo. Although sold nowadays in packages and fermented in climate-controlled rooms using commercially-cultivated mold, natto is still big in Japan, where over 220,000 tons of the stuff is consumed per year. Of the two main varieties, the most popular is called "Itohiki-" or "pulls the thread-" natto because of its stringy consistency (the other type, "Shio natto," is made with a different mold called "koji"). Anyway, natto's cheesy texture and taste have made it notorious and hard for some Westerners to swallow, which is too bad. Like tofu, tempeh, miso, and other foods made from funky soybeans, this so-called "meat of the field" is high in protein, calcium, iron, phosphorus, fiber, vitamins B12 and B2 (riboflavin), and has been shown to fight cancer and lower cholesterol. Additionally, natto contains unique enzymes like nattokinase and pyrazine that seem to break up blood clots, although these chemicals tend to get destroyed during cooking. This is fine by true fans of natto, who typically eat it "raw" with rice for breakfast, often mixed with egg, hot mustard, and/or green onions. Its strong aroma and flavor also make natto a popular condiment.

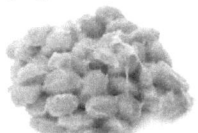

http://www.foodsubs.com

NETTLES

More than 500 species of nettles in the family *Urticaceae* can be found throughout the world, in both tropical and temperate climates. Anyone who has accidentally brushed against a common stinging nettle plant knows that its tiny hairs are an irritant to the skin, producing a burning, stinging rash. This reaction is mild compared to an East Indian species, which produces a prickling sensation followed by burning heat and pain similar to lockjaw that lasts for many hours or even days. The effects of another species, *U. urentissima*, can last for a whole year, and the reaction is said to cause death is some cases. Significantly less poisonous, the common nettle plant found in this climate, *Urtica dioica*, grows to be two to three feet tall and has small flowers and tiny hairs on their dark green leaves and stems. These hairs contain a compound of formic acid, histamine, serotonin, acetylcholine, and 5-hydroxytryptamine, a combination responsible for the stinging reaction, which is lost with cooking or drying. Historically, nettle roots have been used to make ale, nettle juice as a substitute for rennet to make cheese, and nettle fibers to weave durable cloth. In Scotland, a suitor may place nettles between the sheets of a loved one's bed to ensure reciprocal affection or a positive answer to a proposal. Used as a folk remedy for centuries, nettles have expectorant, antispasmodic, diuretic, astringent, and tonic actions and are collected before flowering to treat allergies, asthma, and chronic rheumatism. Nettles are rich in chlorophyll, and young cooked nettle shoots are an excellent source of beta carotene, vitamin C, vitamin E and minerals, including silica.

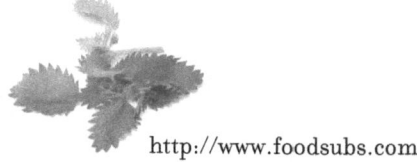

http://www.foodsubs.com

NONI

With luscious foliage, creamy-white flowers and fruits that turn from green to yellow to white, this tropical tree is considered one of the more beautiful on the South Pacific islands, its native home. The plant is prized primarily, though, for its near-magical healing powers. In Polynesia, in fact, noni has been the most important medicinal plant for over 2000 years, used to cure infections, diabetes, high blood pressure, arthritis, hemmorrhaging, coughing, malaria, and other ailments, and to promote general well-being. In the Carribbean, noni is called the Pain Killer Tree and is used to break fevers and heal broken bones. It's known as *nonu* in Samoa, *nono* in Tahiti, *nhan* in Southeast Asia, *mengkudu* in Malasia, and is big among Australian Aborigines and in the Philippines. All parts of the plant – roots, bark, leaves, and seeds – have been used to treat one thing or another, but noni's most popular (and probably most potent) healer is its potato-sized fruits, which contain a chemical that a Dr. Ralph Heinicke, who analyzed noni 4 or 5 years ago, named "xeronine." This small alkaloid seems to regulate the rigidity and shape of proteins, increasing a cell's ability to absorb and use nutrients. It regenerates tissue, inhibits tumors, strengthens the immune system, and has been shown to neutralize highly poisonous substances. Noni actually contains very little xeronine, but it's chock full of "proxeronine" and an enzyme called "proxeronase," which combine in the small intestine to form xeronine. Since 1995, noni juice has been sold commercially by Morinda, a company named after noni's genus (the species name is *citrifolia*), who has a contract with Tahiti to harvest the fruit from the jungle. The juice supposedly tastes terrible by itself, but is quite palatable when combined with other juices. For maximum effect, it is usually taken on an empty stomach, because tummy acids tend to wipe out noni's crucial enzymes.

NORI

Seaweeds have been enjoyed by Asians for ages, but are only starting to catch on in the US. These hardy plants are packed with vitamins, minerals, and protein, have almost no fat, and help remove radiactive heavy elements from the body. Nori, also called "sea lettuce," is a red algae that's usually dried and flattened into paper-thin sheets that are used to make sushi rolls. A different but closely related species called "laver" is still big in Scotland and Wales, where it's processed into "black butter" or used to make a kind of bread. Anyway, nori has as much protein as meat and eggs, as much vitamin A by weight as carrots, plenty of vitamin C, some of the Bs, and lots of calcium and iron. It's also thought to lower cholesterol and have antibiotic qualities. The words "sushi nori" or "yakinori" on the package means it's been pre-toasted; otherwise, you can just pass it over a gas flame until it turns from purple-black to greenish brown. In addition to its role as a wrapper for rice and fish, it can shredded and added to soups, bean and grain salads, or crumbled onto greens or even popcorn.

Nori sheets

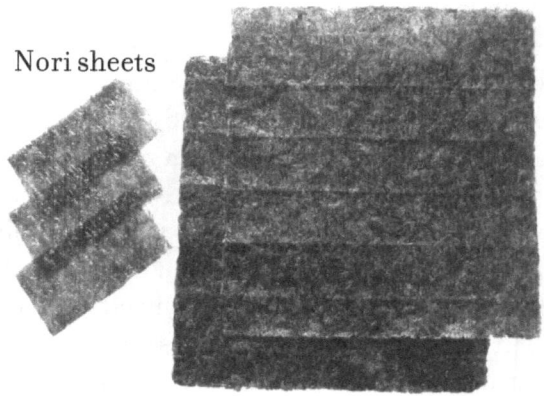

http://rikaty.files.wordpress.com

NUTRITIONAL YEAST

is a single celled fungi, *Saccharomyce cerevisiae*, and an easily digestible food supplement that is grown on a mineral-enriched molasses solution. Unlike live yeast that is used in baking, a nutritional yeast culture is pasteurized at the end of the growth period to kill the yeast. This prevents the microorganism from continuing to grow in the user's intestines and using up the body's nutrients. Egyptian records document the earliest use of yeast around 1550 BCE, but nutritional yeast is recent on the culinary time line, making its way into diets within the past few decades. Nutritional yeast contains 18 amino acids (all the essential amino acids are in there) and 15 minerals, including chromium or the Glucose Tolerance Factor, which helps regulate blood sugar and is important for diabetics and people with low blood sugar. Rich in B-complex vitamins, nutritional yeast is a valuable supplement within the vegetarian population. This yeast has a yellow-gold color (because of the riboflavin content), comes in either powder or flake form, and tastes somewhat cheesy. Sprinkle nutritional yeast on rice, vegetables, and popcorn, add a teaspoon to sauces, gravies, breadings, and baked goods, and put some in your scrambled tofu recipe. You can even give your dog or cat nutritional yeast to supplement good nutrition and to promote a healthy coat.

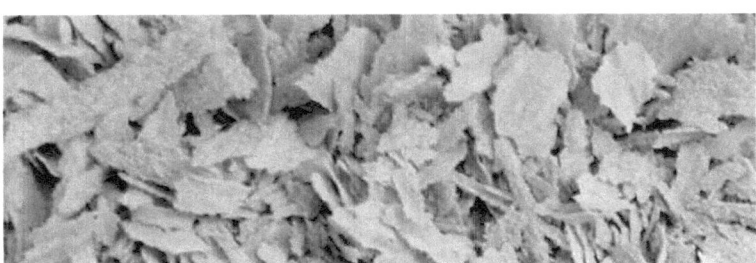

http://www.all-creatures.org

are by-products from the production of soy milk. Okara is the pulp left after the liquid (milk) has been strained out of ground, cooked soybeans. It doesn't have as much protein as the whole bean, but what it does have is of a higher quality. It is sometimes consumed to enrich the milk of nursing mothers. Alone it tastes a little like coconut, or is sometimes combined with spices to make soy sausage (aka soysage). Yuba, which has been eaten by vegetarian Buddhist monks for centuries, is the layer that forms on top of hot soymilk as it cools. It has been described as "the condensed essence or elixir of the soymilk's flavor and nutrients," being high in protein and minerals. Fresh yuba is tough to come by in this country, but you might be able to find it dried, either in flat sheets called "bean curd sheets" or "bean curd skins," or in rolls called "bamboo yuba" or "bean curd sticks." Both kinds need to be soaked in water before use, the sheets for about 30 minutes and the ropes for a few hours. It can then be sliced and used in stir fries or light soups.

Yuba

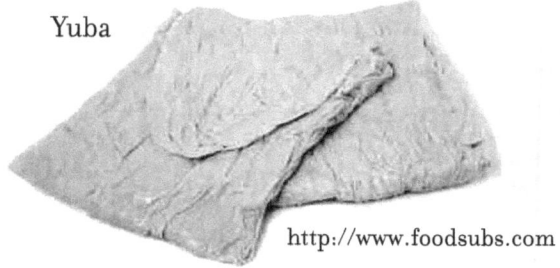

http://www.foodsubs.com

OKRA

is a vegetable that comes from a large, African plant in the same family as hibiscus and cotton. It was brought to this continent a few centuries back by Ethiopian slaves, although it name is supposedly a variation on "nkruma," a West African word. Anyway, the long, tapered, fruit of the plant is also called "lady finger." When cooked, it releases sticky stuff that thickens up soups and stews. In the South, it's sometimes called "gumbo" because it's the star of that famous dish. It can also be eaten raw, or cooked with other vegetables like onions, tomatoes, peppers, or eggplant, which it sort of tastes like. Folks who don't like its squishy quality might soak it in salted water, roll it in cornmeal and fry it; it's also popular pickled. In Indian cooking, "bhindi" is usually sautéed with currry, cumin, coriander, turmeric, and other nice spices. Chinese okra, by the way, is a different food altogether. Okra is low in calories and sodium, high in vitamins A , C, and B1 (thiamin), and provides a goodly dose of magnesium.

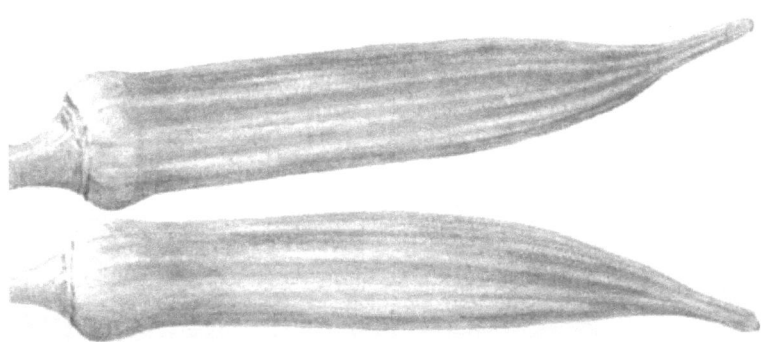

http://oldvegiepatch1972.googlepages.com

OREGANO

The Greek word "origanos" means "joy of the mountains," probably because that's where this hardy perennial tends to grow wild. For ages, peoples of the Mediterranean have dried and crushed the green or gray-green leaves of *Oreganum vulgare* and sprinkled them on oiled flatbread and other foods to add flavor and promote vitality. These days, commercial oregano is grown mostly in Greece and Moroccco, and winds up most frequently in Mexican, Italian, and yes, Greek dishes. The stuff we Americans use is usually not real oregano, but either Spanish thyme (sometimes labeled "Moroccan oregano"), or Mexican sage ("Mexican oregano"). Unfortunately, both of these close relatives lack some of flavor and potency of wild oregano, said to be rich in vitamins C, E, A, and B3, calcium, iron, potassium, zinc and chlorophyll. Oregano's distinct taste and aroma come from its essential oil, which is being touted by people like Dr. Cass Igram as a powerful medicine containing the above nutrients plus thymol and carvacol, compounds that fight bacteria, fungi (such as those that cause athletes foot), viruses (like herpes), and other microbes that bring about hayfever and allergies (without promoting resistant strains like synthetic antibiotics do). The oil is also said to kick asthma, bronchitis, colds and flu, to work as an antiseptic, a pain killer, and a natural preservative. It can be taken internally (a few drops under the tongue) or applied on the outside to scratches and other boo-boos. The camphorous-smelling oil is also sometimes used in soaps and perfumes.

PARSLEY

Use of this biennial plant goes back to ancient Greece, where it was put on the heads of victorious athletes and on tombs and graves because of its association with Archemorous, a heralder of death. Ancient Romans ate it to prevent drunkenness, since apparently they hadn't figured out that sobriety could just as easily be achieved by not drinking alcohol. Today, the plant's frilly leaves are popular as a food flavorer and salad ingredient in the Mediterranean region, as well as in Europe and the Middle East. In America, parsley sprigs appear frequently as a garnish that most people don't eat, which is unfortunate since they contain a healthful dose of calcium, iron, potassium, vitamins A, C, B_1 (thiamine), and B_2 (riboflavin), plus chloropyll, which gives parsley some of its breath-freshening power. A member of the family that includes carrots, caraway, coriander, celery, and parsnips, *Petroselinum crispum* comes in three main varieties: Curly-leaf (the most common), Italian or broad-leaf (the most flavorful and beloved by cooks), and Hamburg or Dutch parsley, notorious for its white, carrot-shaped, celery-flavored root. Medicinally, the parsley has been used to cleanse the intestinal and urinary tracts and fight asthma, allergies, and bronchitis, while its essential oil has been found to help lower blood pressure. It should not be consumed in any large quantity by expectant mothers.

http://members.tripod.com

PAU D'ARCO

This South American rainforest herb and the large ever-green tree from which it comes also go by the Indian names "Taheebo" and "Ipe Roxo." The Spanish name, "Lapacho Morado," refers to the tree's big, purple flowers which distinguish it from related species that don't quite pack the healing power of *Tabebuia impetiginosa*, which has been used since pre-Incan times to treat everything from internal illnesses like malaria, respiratory problems, colds, flu, infections, arthritis, diabetes, ulcers, to external ailments like athlete's foot, boils, snakebites, and other wounds. Guarani Indians, who called the tree "tajy," which means "to have strength and vigor," thought of it as the "giver of life" and used its bark as their main medicine. Lapacho has been studied scientifically since the late 1800s, but mostly in this century by Dr. Theodoro Meyer, an Argentinian who touted it as a practical cure-all. It caught on in the '60s in Brazil, where it has become a standard anti-cancer treatment, shown to relieve pain, shrink tumors, and even cause remission of the dread disease, with no side effects other than occasional nausea for first-time users (believed to be caused by the herb's general detoxifying action). Pau d'arco has been gaining popularity in the US since the early '80s, mostly as an energy and immunity booster and a possible treatment for HIV. The herb has been found to contain over 20 active ingredients, the most potent being *lapochol*, which was actually discovered way back in 1884 and synthesized in 1927. This phytochemical, which seems to oxygenate red blood cells in the bone marrow, is concentrated mostly in the inner bark or phloem of the lapacho tree, which, unfortunately, is also prized for its heavy, durable wood. In fact, a lot of bulk pau d'arco is stuff that's been stripped off at the sawmill, which means it may contain the bitter outer bark, the actual wood, or may even be from a different tree (like mahogany, which has a similar smell and color). For this reason, it's a safer bet to buy the herb in capsule or extract form.

Pau d'arco bark shavings

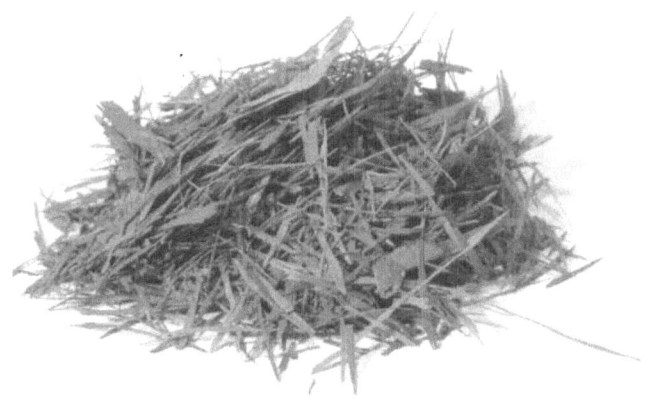

https://www.mysticearth.net

PIGEON PEAS,

also known as "gandules," "congo peas" or "no-eyed peas," come from a vigorous, yellow-flowered plant that hails from Africa or maybe India, depending on who you ask. Whatever their origin, about 80% of them are nowadays grown on the subcontinent, where they tend to wind up in *dahl*. They're also popular in the Caribbean, where they go good with rice, sometimes in place of black-eyed peas in the famous New Year's dish, Hoppin' John. They're semi-popular in Latin America and the southern US, although the pigeon pea is not a big cash crop in this here country. These high-protein legumes grow in twisted, fuzzy pods (also edible) and are about the size of your garden-variety peas, but with a yellowy-gray hue and a sweet flavor. They're usually harvested dry, and sold split or canned. The pigeon pea plant is sometimes put along the sides of houses, because its poisonous roots can protect against moles and termites. It's also handy because of its ability to enrich the soil by adding nitrogen.

To make a simple dahl, soak 2 cups of gandules for 20 minutes, put them into 1.5 quarts of water with 6 cloves, 6 cardamoms, 1/2 tsp peppercorns, 1 tsp turmeric, salt, and a couple bay leaves, and boil for 20 minutes. Chop and sautée an onion with 4 cloves garlic and a diced green chili or two, then mix with the beans and simmer.

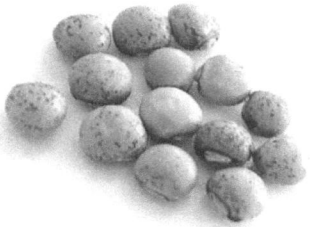

http://www.victoryseeds.com

PLANTAINS

When Americans say "banana," they're usually referring to the yellow fruit, a dessert variety called the *Gros Michel*, which makes up less than 15% of all bananas in the world. The other 85% are actually grown and eaten locally in the tropics as a staple food. One of the most common subspecies is the plantain, also known as *ndizi* or *pisang*, which probably originated in what's now Malaysia, traveled with migrants over to Madagascar, then on to Africa and beyond. While resembling sweet, yellow bananas, plantains are bigger, harder to peel, and too starchy to be eaten raw until fully ripened to black. Young, green plantains have the texture of potatoes, and are sometimes boiled and mashed like spuds. At any stage, plantains can also be baked, broiled, grilled, sautéed, deep fried, roasted, or dried and ground into flour. They're high in carbos, potassium, magnesium, fiber, and vitamin C. The juice of the fruit allegedly acts as an antidote against snake venom, while the plant's huge leaves can be cut into strips and woven into mats or bags, or used (whole) as thatching for roofs or platters on which to serve a tasty meal of rice and plantains.

To make a baked version, peel a few plantains by first cutting off the ends, then making a slit along the inside curve. Slice the fruit lengthwise into flat strips, place on a baking sheet, sprinkle on some lemon juice and cumin or curry, and bake at 325° or so until browned on the edges but still a little soft in the middle.

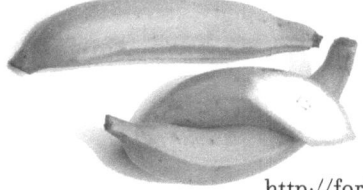

http://forkyou.files.wordpress.com

POMEGRANATE

Indigenous to the Near East (perhaps Persia), the spiny, deciduous bush (or small tree) from which this fruit comes, *Punica granatum*, is unique enough to be the only member of its genus, which is the only member of its botanical family (*Punicaceae*). The one-of-a-kind fruit (or berry) itself, with its red-brown, leathery skin surrounding hundreds of magenta seeds embedded in a pinkish pulp, has a long and sordid history, going way back to ancient Phoenicia and Greece, where it was associated with abundance and fertility. It was mentioned in Homer's *Odyssey* and cited in the Old Testament as a fruit of the Promised Land (it may have even been the one that Adam and Eve ingested). Once known as "Malum punicum" or "apple of Carthage," the fruit was a favorite of wise guys like King Solomon and Mohammed, the latter of whom claimed that it "purges the system of envy and hatred." In Ayurveda, the rootbark of *dadima* has been known to purge the body of other nasties, such as worms, dysentery, and ulcers, while its fruit and rind have been used against inflammation, and its juice for promoting digestion and purifying the blood. Apparently the easiest way to access the Vitamin C, potassium, and fiber in a *pomme garnette* ("seeded apple" in French) is to score its thin skin and break it into quarters, which can be submerged in water, causing the seeds to sink and the flesh to float. Of course, the sweet-tart seeds can also be picked out by hand, as long as you don't mind your fingers turning bright red from the juice, which is also capable of dyeing clothing and rugs. Pomegranates are sometimes used to make grenadine, a light syrup often added to sweets, soft drinks, and cocktails, as well as the thicker pomegranate molasses (*dibs rumman* in Arabic), which appears in Mediterranean dishes like *muhammara*, a dip that also includes peppers and walnuts.

PRIMROSE OIL

Evening Primrose is a perrennial plant with 4-petaled, yellow flowers that has grown in North America for over 70,000 years. Native peoples used to collect its cylindrical pods and use the itty bitty seeds as food and to make a painkiller. In the 1600s, the plant was brought to Europe, where it was called "king's cure-all." These days, the oil pressed from Primrose seeds is used to treat maybe not *all*, but lots of ailments: arthritis, diabetes, chronic fatigue, heart disease, high blood pressure, even multiple sclerosis. It has been shown to cause cholesterol levels to drop 31% in just 3 months, and is the most common and effective treatment for PMS, which is nowadays thought to be caused not by a hormonal imbalance but by a nutritional deficiency. The oil's magical ingredients are those essential fatty acids you've heard so much about, especially one called Gamma Linoleic Acid. GLA helps form "prostoglandins," which regulate blood pressure, heartbeat, and other natural functions; it's good for your brain, your skin, and your circulation. Primrose oil has slightly less of this special acid than flaxseed oil and borage oil, but what it has is apparently more "bioactive" and user friendly.

Evening primrose

http://www.oaklandnaturepreserve.org

PSYLLIUM

This fibrous foodstuff comes from the dried seed husks of *plantago psyllium*, a.k.a. blond or Indian psyllium, a relative of the plantain. In days of yore, psyllium seed, also called "fleaseed," was used to treat ulcers and stomach problems. As one of the world's best sources of roughage, psyllium is nowadays often added to breakfast cereals, and is the active ingredient in laxatives like Metamucil and Fiberall. The source of psyllium's gut-cleansing power is mucilage, a water-soluble fiber that turns to gel as it passes through your plumbing. Since mucilage expands as it soaks up water, psyllium has been used as an appetite supressant, but it has also been shown to reduce bad cholesterol and thereby lower the risk of heart disease. At the very least, psyllium will keep you regular, which is important because constipation, in addition to being highly uncomfortable, is the sign of a toxic body and can lead to more serious problems like hemmorrhoids, gallstones, and colon cancer, which is caused by nasty stuff hanging out in the lower bowel for too long. Psyllium can be bought in seed form or in tablets. It should be taken with lots of liquid, and perhaps not at all by people prone to allergies.

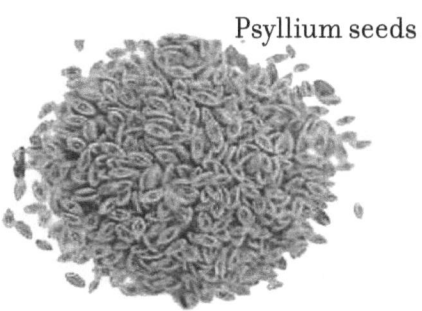

Psyllium seeds

http://product-image.tradeindia.com

PUMPKIN

is a winter squash from the same family as gourds, melons, zucchini, and cucumbers. It supposedly hails from Asia, but has been known on this continent for ages. In fact, the word squash comes from the Iroquois word "isquotersquash," which means something like "eaten raw," which Native Americans used to do. The flowers that grow on squash vines are also edible, and were used in cooking and ritual, especially in the southwest. Like most of its relatives, pumpkins are high in complex carbos. They're a great source of beta carotene (vitamin A), an antioxidant that protects against cancer and blood vessel damage, and are high in fiber and low in calories. Jack-o'-lanterns were invented in Ireland and used to be carved from turnips, potatoes, or rutabagas (pumpkins are an American thing). They're named after a miserly, drunken fella who outwitted the devil to live a long life. When he died, Satan gave him a burning coal which he stuck in a hollow tuber to light his eternal wanderings between heaven and hell. After carving, pumpkin seeds can be spread on a baking sheet and roasted for 45 minutes at 375°. These seeds are high in protein, phosphorus, and magnesium, and have more iron than any other seed. They've even been used as a treatment for prostate cancer. They're a little oily, but you have to eat about 150 seeds to get one ounce of fat, which is unsaturated anyway, and they sure beat Snickers and Twizzlers as a healthy Halloween snack. Speaking of healthy, here's a recipe for pumpkin pie filling:

Blend 4 cups cooked pumpkin with 1 cup vanilla soymilk, 1/3 cup maple syrup, and a pinch of sea salt. Add 2 tbsp agar-agar, simmer for 5 minutes, then stir in 1 tbsp kuzu (diluted with water) to thicken. Remove from heat and add 1 tsp vanilla and 3/4 tsp allspice.

QUINOA

This ancient "supergrain," an old favorite of the Incas, prefers to grow in high-altitude regions like the Andes in Peru. Technically, this "grain that grows where grass will not" is not a grain at all, but the fruit of an herby plant related to chard and spinach. Whatever they are, quinoa's little, millet-like granules certainly are nutritious, containing a copius amount of protein, lots of fiber, more vitamins and minerals than just about any other grain, and chemicals like phytic acid that may fight cancer and high cholesterol. This impressive profile, by the way, has earned quinoa a special recognition by the United Nations Food and Agricultural Organization, for whatever that's worth. Before cooking quinoa, you may want to give it a rinsing to get rid of a bitter chemical called saponin said to act as the plant's natural insect repellant. Using twice as much water as grain, boil for about 15 minutes, let the stuff sit for awhile, then fluff it with a fork. Cooked grains are 3 or 4 times bigger than uncooked grains, and have cute, little tails that impart a slight crunch. Quinoa lends itself well to everything from soups to desserts.

To make a strikingly colorful salad, mix quinoa with grated beets, then add lemon juice, fresh, chopped parsley, scallions, and salt to taste.

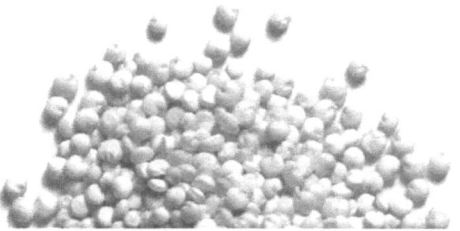

http://www.dkimages.com

RAPINI

also called broccoli rabe, raab, or rape, is a vegetable related to cabbage and turnips that looks kind of like regular broccoli. Unlike its sibling, though, it's known and grown for its large leaves rather than its immature flower buds, although it does have its own little florets on the end of long stems, which can also be eaten after peeling. Rapini is big with people in Italy, but is unfortunately enjoyed mostly by farm animals in this country, perhaps because of its strong, tangy flavor. The greens can be made less bitter by dropping them in salted, boiling water for a few minutes, or by sprinkling them with red wine vinegar after cooking. A quick and popular way to fix rapini is by sautéeing in olive oil with garlic and red pepper flakes, then tossing into pasta. This cruciferous vegetable has very little sodium and few calories, lots of potassium and vitamins A, C. and K.

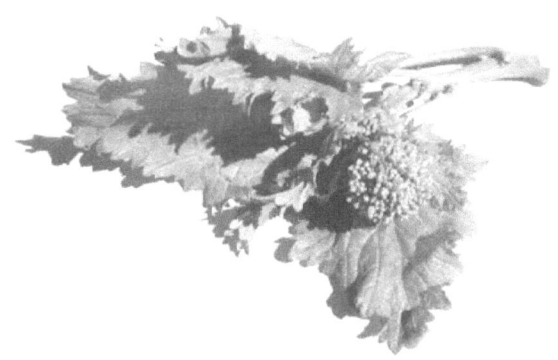

http://www.gourmetsleuth.com

111

REISHI

is the Japanese name for *ganoderma lucidum*, a type of mushroom originally used in China, where it's called Ling Zhi, or "spirit plant." A wise guy named Seng Nong, who wrote the oldest known Chinese medical text, classified over 365 herbs and other natural things and ranked this fungus as #1, believing it to extend life. Once upon a time, it was so rare that only emporors ate it, but since 1971 it's been cultivated artificially. Modern science has found that this 'shroom has antibacterial and anticancer effects, lowers cholesterol, and helps with high blood pressure and clotting. Its adaptogens help the body deal with stress, its antioxidants destroy those pesky "free radicals" that damage cell walls and proteins and promote aging, and its highly active polysaccharides (sugar chains) and terpenoids boost the immune system. Nutritionally, it's got vitamins, minerals, and complete proteins. Reishi comes in a variety of colors depending on how it's grown, but red is apparently the most potent. The mushroom itself is hard, woody, and mostly indigestible, so its goodness is usually steeped out in tea, or extracted and sold in powdered or tablet form.

To fix an elixir, simmer a teaspoon of chopped, dried Reishi and a few slices of thinly-sliced ginger in one cup of water for 10 minutes.

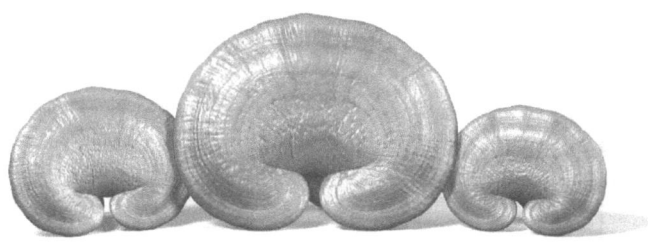

http://solarisfarma.com

RICE BRAN OIL

The difference between whole-grain (brown) rice and white rice is bran, the outer layer of the grain which happens to be the most nutritious part, containing lots of vitamin B6, iron, phosphorus, magnesium, potassium, and fiber. During the processing of white rice, sadly, this goodness gets removed and used as animal feed, fertilizer, or just tossed out. Gladly, some food companies have taken to rescuing this "by-product" and using it to make stuff like rice bran cereal, rice bran milk, or the increasingly popular rice bran oil. Apparently over 1/3 of all Japanese restaurants have switched to this healthful oil, which has been shown to reduce cholesterol levels up to 30% when ingested regularly. Strangely, even though rice bran oil has more saturated fat than olive and corn oils, it still has a greater cholesterol-lowering effect (in general, saturated fats tend to raise cholesterol levels, while unsaturated fats lower them). Scientists suspect this is because rice bran oil contains a unique substance called "oryzanol," as well as other fancy, fat-busting chemicals like tocopherols and tocotrienols. Rice bran oil also contains plenty of vitamin E, which is good for the cardiovascular system, as well as "Coenzyme Q10" (CoQ), another nutrient needed for a healthy ticker. Other general benefits of this oil are its ability to help the body retain calcium and fight off kidney stones. Rice bran oil's delicate flavor and high smoke point make it a splendid choice for cooking and frying, or as an ingredient in dressing.

ROOIBOS

In the mountains northwest of Capetown in South Africa grows *Aspalathus linearis*, a member of the legume family which turns from dark green to red-brown, earning itself the nickname "red bush" (Rooibos in Africaan). At the beginning of this century, a popular "red tea" was marketed and made from the nettle-like leaves and fine stems of a few wild subspecies, but in 1930 a certain Dr. Nortier began cultivating the "Nortieria" variety from which all Rooibos now comes. This herb has been found to contain the highest concentration of the antioxidant "super-oxide bismutase" (SOD) of any plant on the planet, including green tea. The free-radical-busting power of Rooibos is backed up by other antioxidants like vitamins C and A, chlorophyll, and a bio-flavonoid called "quercetin," which improves circulation by increasing capillary strength. To boot, Rooibos is packed with calcium, iron, magnesium, potassium, and fluoride, contains no unhealthy, nerve-frazzling caffeine and is low in tannins, substances found in non-herbal teas which interfere with the absorption of iron and protein. Rooibos tea reportedly relieves stomach cramps, asthma, hayfever, heartburn and hangovers, boosts energy, and cures colic and insomnia in infants. Applied externally, it improves the complexion and helps with eczema and itching. With its deep red color and earthy but naturally sweet taste, Rooibos tea is great hot or on the rocks (try some mixed with fruit juice or ginger ale), and can even be used as a colorful and nutritious base for soups and sauces.

is a viscuous, milky substance produced in the glands of worker bees. Little baby larvae are fed this goo for just a few days, but the queen bee, who is not genetically superior to the rest of the bees, eats it her whole life, enabling her to get 50% bigger than the workers, become a reproductive dynamo able to lay twice her own weight in eggs per day, and live 5-7 years instead of about 6 weeks like her servants. Humans who eat royal jelly probably won't get huge and extra fertile, but it does seem to impart energy and royal health. It contains 35% protein, all the essential aminos, vitamins A thru E, and lots of minerals like calcium and iron. It's nature's best source for the B vitamin pantothenic acid, which is good for stress, fatigue, and arthritis, and contains acetylcholine, a conductor of nerve impulses. It's good on the skin and is reported to have anti-bacterial and anti-aging effects. Other bee products that are good for (non-vegan) people include pollen, which has loads of protein, aminos, and vitamins, purifies the blood, and may fight cancer; and propolis, a waxy substance that bees get from the buds of trees and bushes and spread all over the hive to protect it from contamination. In humans, it acts as a natural antibiotic that destroys only bad bacteria, unlike unnatural antibiotics which kill good bacteria while they're at it.

http://www.arihanaricilik.com

SAFFRON

When the *Crocus sativus* begins to bloom in October and November, skilled workers take to the fields to strip away the petals of this small purple plant and pluck out their three yellow-orange stigmas by hand. An experienced and perseverant picker can de-stigma about 10-12,000 flowers a day, which will yield a scanty 2 ounces after drying. Moreover, the flowering period lasts only 10 days, so such assiduous effort is necessary during the bloom. After being picked and dried in the sun (or by artificial heat), the one-inch long stigmas are ready to be packaged, labeled, and shipped under the name of saffron. This toilsome process explains saffron's reputation as the world's most expensive spice. Although saffron has also been used to dye cloth and body oil and to make medicines, today this pungent, aromatic spice is used primarily to make tea and flavor and color foods like bouillabaisse, risotto Milanese, and paella. Saffron can be found in both powdered form (beware of fillers) and thread form (crush before using), and luckily for the consumer a little bit goes a long way. Sources say the saffron from Spain is the best, because there are higher levels of essential pigments and oils. However, better quality also mean higher prices - up to four times more for Spanish saffron.

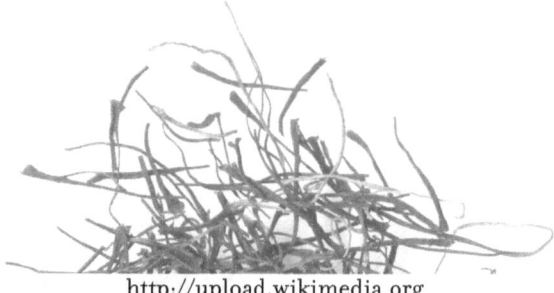

http://upload.wikimedia.org

SAGE

The garden variety of this herb, known as White Sage, True Sage, or – more officially – *Salvia officinalis*, is native to southern Europe, but now grows in lots of other places like Russia, America, and especially the Mediterranean. Its popularity as a medicinal herb is apparent in its genus name (which means "to save" in Latin), and in an old Arabian phrase: "Why should a man die while he has sage in his garden?" Throughout the ages, sage's skinny, blue-grey leaves have been infused and used to ward off coughs and colds, improve circulation, digestion, and memory, and to help concieve babies. They've also been chewed or otherwise softened to make poultices for cleaning and healing wounds and bug bites. As a food, sage has A, C, and B complex vitamins, calcium, potassium, and a slightly camphorous taste (owing to its membership in the mint family) that's earned it a place on many a spice rack. It's frequently a flavoring for fatty meats, but does make appearances in kinder, gentler, healthier foods, including Middle Eastern salads. Referred to by the old Romans as "herba sacra," sage is sometimes "smudged" or burned ritually for protection, cleansing, or to impart wisdom or prosperity, while its fragrant essential oil often ends up in liquor and perfumes.

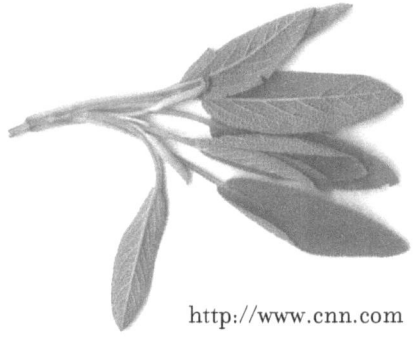

http://www.cnn.com

ST. JOHN'S WORT

In Olde English, the word "wort" means "root" or "plant," while Saint John refers to the guy who baptized Jesus. In medieval times, folks in Europe, believing the plant had magical powers, would stick it under pillows to influence dreams, hang it above doorways to keep out evil spirits, and stuff it into the mouths of suspected witches in order to get a confession (albeit a muffled one). The bushy herb's yellow flowers, which blossom around the summer solstice, would be picked on St. John's day (June 25th) and soaked in olive oil to produce a red anointing oil called "the blood of Christ." The red pigment comes from the herb's main active ingredient, hypericin, a chemical which inhibits the re-uptake of certain neurotransmitters like seratonin, resulting in more of these brain chemicals, causing mood elevation, leading to incredible demand for the herb over the past few years. Indeed, sales of St. John's Wort, which has been used for centuries to cure "melancholia," increased 3900% from 1995 to 1998. Called "nature's Prozac," the herb is used to treat the majority of cases of depression in Germany, where it outsells its synthetic competitor 7 to 1, and has become quite popular in the US. By now most people have heard about St. John's Wort's psychological effects, but fewer are aware that it's also been used to relieve arthritis, muscle spasms, menstrual cramps, and pain in general. It's also good for the guts, fights ulcers and tumors, and may inhibit the growth of viruses like HIV. Most users report no side effects, though some get an upset tummy or become sensitive to sunburn (fortunately, oil made from St. John's Wort also heals the skin). Unfortunately, it may not be so good for pregnant women (it was once thought to bring about abortions) or children, and since there are no official standards of quality for commercial St. John's Wort, its potency varies greatly from brand to brand.

SARSAPARILLA

Given that the Spanish word *sarza* means "bramble," and *parilla* means "vine," it shouldn't surprise you to learn that almost all species of this perennial grow as a vine with prickly stems. Most varieties are also used to treat various ailments, such as those of the liver (like jaundice, hepatitis, and gout) or the joints (arthritis, rheumatism, and inflammation), although the most common uses of sarsaparilla throughout the world seem to be for skin problems and syphilis. In Persia, the plant's young shoots are eaten as a vegetable, while in parts of southern China its woody vines are woven into baskets. American sarsaparilla, a.k.a. Wild Licorice or Rabbit Root, was used by native peoples like the Cree, who taught white settlers to make a beverage from the plant's roots, which contain saponins responsible for sarsaparilla's sweet flavor and foaminess. In the 1800s, "root beer" was made with with alcohol, which seemed to increase the drink's medicinal effects, such as increasing the "perspiratory functions of the skin" and "imparting tone and vigor to debilitated constitutions." These days, most root beer is made with artificial sweeteners and flavors, contributing neither the medicinal benefits of sarsaparilla nor the calcium, iron, manganese, potassium, and vitamins A, B, C and D it contains. Fortunately, sarsaparilla's goodness is available in tablet form.

Root

http://www.us.luluherbal.com

SCHIZANDRA

Also spelled "schisandra," this creeping, thorny bush from the magnolia family is native to northern China and Manchuria, where ancient hunter-gatherers once used the plant's small, wrinkly, red berries as a staple food. These fruits, called "wu wei tzu," or "many-flavored berry," supposedly contain all of traditional Chinese medicine's basic tastes: sweet, sour, salty, pungent, and bitter. Anyway, in 2697 BCE, Huang Ti included schizandra in his "Yellow Emperor's Classic of Internal Medicine," praising its ability to fight ailments of the liver, lungs, and digestive region. It was also thought to boost sexual energy, which made it a favorite of subsequent emperor types. During WWII, the berries were used by Russian fighter pilots to relieve eye fatigue as well as general fatigue, as they contain a mild stimulant. Modern studies reveal that *Schizanra chenensis* does improve the eye's ability to adapt to darkness, as well as the liver's ability to ward off damage using chemicals called "lignans." Schizandra has also been shown to increase stamina, combat motion sickness, and balance blood sugar levels. It may also help lower cholesterol and high blood pressure by improving circulation. Schizandra's main claim to fame is that it contains "adaptogens," magical chemicals also found in foods like ginseng and reishi mushrooms that increase the body's ability to resist disease and the effects of stress. Usually sold as an extract in tablet form, schizandra has no major side effects, although it's not recommended for pregnant women.

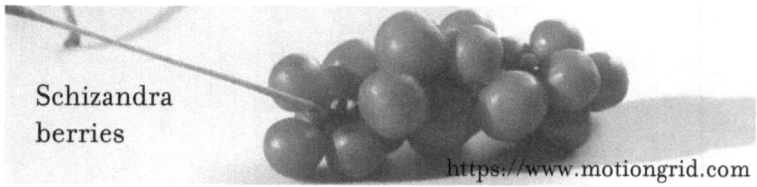

Schizandra
berries

https://www.motiongrid.com

SEITAN,

sometimes sold simply as "wheat gluten," is a mild-tasting starchless gluten made with tamari soy sauce. Because of its hearty, substantial, somewhat chewy texture, it is often used in "mock meat" dishes and soups, and also appears frequently in spicy sautées and curries because of its tendency to soak up seasonings. Seitan is high in protein, calcium, and niacin (vitamin B3).

To make seitan, mix 4 cups whole wheat flour with enough water to make a dough. Knead for 5 minutes, then place in a bowl, cover with cold water, and leave for 10 minutes. Replace the cold water with warm, and knead in the water to remove most of the starch and bran. Knead the sticky gluten for 2 minutes in a strainer, under cold water, then hot, alternating 4 or 5 times until all the starch and bran are washed out. Cut into chunks, boil, and slice into strips. Simmer in water with 1/3 cup tamari, 1 tbsp. ginger juice, and a strip of kombu, for 25 to 40 minutes.

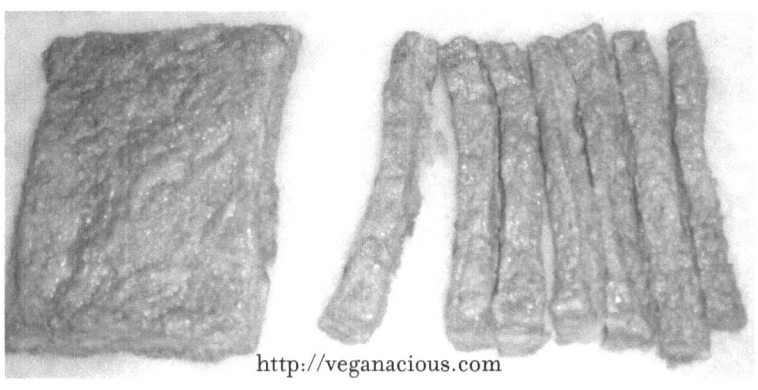

http://veganacious.com

SESAME OIL,

also called gingelly or benne oil, is a pale yellowish oil that's probably one of the best, along with maybe cold-pressed corn oil, to use for general cooking. It's been used for centuries in Africa, and, of course, in the Orient. It's pretty popular in hot climates because, unlike other oils, it contains a magical natural ingredient called sesamol that keeps it from going bad in the heat, and consuming rancid oil causes a loss of vitamins in the body, which is bad. With any oil, cold pressed is best, because heat used during other processing methods produces peroxides that destroy the vitamin E. Because sesame seeds have no husks, a single cold pressing is about all it takes to extract the oil, which has lots of E and is about 40% linoleic acid, an essential nutrient. Certain oils, like safflower and sunflower, have more vitamin E and a higher percentage of linoleic, but, because of hard husks, it's tougher to extract these oils without using big machines and crazy chemicals. Dark or "Oriental" sesame oil is made from roasted sesame seeds. It's thicker and has a stronger smell and taste than regular sesame oil, but it loses its flavor as it gets hotter, and burn easily, so be careful when using it to cook. Try using it to sautée some snow peas with a little ginger. It can also be used as a condiment or flavoring for soups, salads, stir fries and such.

SHIITAKE

(she-ta-kay): These mushrooms grow on old oak logs, mostly in Japan, where they used be eaten only by royal types and were called the "king of mushrooms." They were also called "elixir of life" because of their supposed ability to slow down aging and provide lots of "vital energy" (wink wink). Modern Japanese people still eat them with almost every meal and even give them as gifts. Until 1972, it was illegal to import shiitakes into this country because important people got the Latin name, *lentinus edodes*, confused with a different species that destroys railroad ties. As it turns out, shiitakes are not only harmless to railroad ties, but quite good for humans. They have almost twice the protein of most vegetables (between 15 and 35%), lots of fiber and enzymes (they grow really fast), ample B vitamins, and no fat or cholesterol. In fact, a chemical in shiitake called eritadenine even reduces cholesterol and lowers blood pressure. Another substance, lentinum, is an immune booster and stimulates growth hormones. Like most mushrooms, shiitakes are alkaline and help indigestion. They're also said to be good for the flu. Shiitakes are fragrant, with a smoky sort of taste and a chewy texture. They are sold either fresh or dried (the dried ones have a fuller flavor), and can then be baked, sautéed, broiled, or stir fried.

To make a soup stock, use 1.5 oz. dried and destemmed, plus 1/2 lb. sliced, fresh shiitake, a sliced leek, 2 chopped celery stalks, 4 cloves chopped garlic, 1/3 cup parsely, 1/2 tsp sage, 1 tsp tamari, and 9 cups of water. Boil, then cover and simmer 45 minutes. Strain out the vegetables, keeping the mushrooms around for other invigorating concoctions.

SHILAJIT

What may be one of the oddest edible items on earth comes from the Himalayan regions of Tibet, Nepal, Bhutan, China, India, and Pakistan. Here, during the summer months, one might discover oozing from cracks in the mountainside tar-like blobs of compacted organic matter and minerals said to have the smell of stale cow's urine. Although the composition of this substance varies from place to place, there are four main types, the most coveted having a prevalence of iron. Anyhow, shilajit (meaning "the conqueror of mountains" in Sanskrit) has been harvested from the hills since before the time of the classic Ayurvedic treatise *Charaka Samhita*, in which it's described as a *rasayana* capable of rejuvenating the immune system and revitalizing the body's core energy. It has ben prescribed for problems of the kidneys, nerves, and lungs, used against disorders like diabetes, jaundice, and epilepsy, and ingested to aid memory retrieval. The most common use of shilajit, however, is as a *yogavahi*, a substance taken with other medicines and herbs to help with their assimilation and enhance their effectiveness. In the 1970s, scientists began studying shilajit to find out whether it comes from fossilized organic material (bitumen) or stuff that has decomposed more recently. They discovered it to be of modern origin, composed mostly of humus (the organic constituent of soil, not the Middle Eastern chickpea dip) and of the hardened resin of local plants such as *Tripholia repens*. Studies have also isolated shilajit's active ingredients as benzoic and fulvic acids, tripertenes, and phenolic lipids, all chemicals that help with transport of nutrients throughout the body. Fortunately, modern science has also developed ways to extract the good stuff from shilajit, which ordinarily must be carefully selected, ground, and purified of any harmful or overabundant minerals.

SORGHUM

Also called "milo," this hardy, drought-resistant grain was domesticated in Sudan about 5,000 years ago from a type of wild grass. It now ranks as either the fourth or fifth most popular grain in the world (after rice, corn, wheat and maybe barley), and tops the list in most of Africa and East Asia. About 80% of it is grown in those parts, where its flour is used in stuff like flatbreads, porridge, and malted drinks. This high-protein grain was brought to the States around 1700 by African slaves, who may have later coined its old name, "guinea corn." The bulk of what's now grown in the US is of the sweet sorghum variety, most of which, sadly, winds up not on store shelves, but in the bellies of farm animals. The rest goes mainly to produce sorghum molasses, made by crushing milo's corn-like stalks and boiling the juice into a syrup. This sweetener is similar to regular, cane molasses in composition (mostly simple sugars) and nutritional benefits (basically none), but a bit more sour in taste.

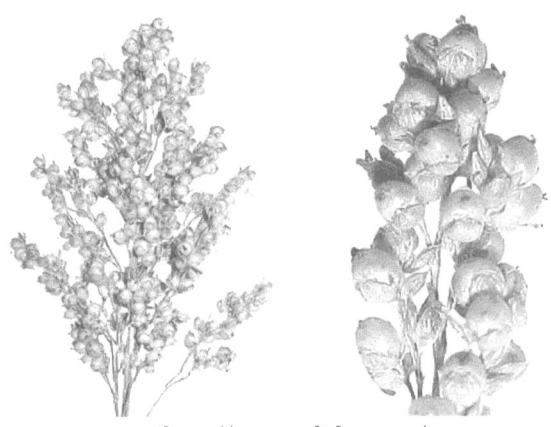

http://www.mdidea.com/

SORREL

is an hardy herb from the buckwheat family that has grown wild in Asia, Europe, and North America for centuries. The garden variety, a.k.a. sour dock or sourgrass, has deep green, spinachy leaves with a lemony zing caused by oxalic acid or "binoxolate of potash," a chemical also found in rhubarb. The leaves get more tangy as the plant gets older, so they're often picked when young. They can then be tossed in salads, shredded in soups (creamy potato with sorrel is a favorite), or puréed in sauces. In France, French sorrel is used to make a green sauce that's usually served with fish and is said to be "good for them that have sicke and feeble stomaches." Caribbean sorrel, related to the hibiscus, has deep red leaves that are used to make a traditional Christmas drink, and give red zinger tea its lovely hue. Sorrel contains lots of vitamins A and C, minerals like calcium, phosphorus, magnesium, and potassium, and is supposedly good for the glands.

To make a sorrel-chive pesto, blend 1 cup chopped sorrel, 3 TB each of parsley and chives, 4 TB each of shallots and pine nuts or almonds, 2-3 grated orange rinds, and 1/4 of a red onion. Add 1 TB dry mustard and a little salt and pepper, then slowly drizzle 3/4 cups of olive oil into the blender to make a smooth and tasty paste.

http://static.howstuffworks.com

SPELT

is a grain that used to be so popular in Germany and in the Old World in general that it was called "the rice of Europe," even though it's not very rice-like. In fact, it's a kissin' cousin of wheat, which is what its grains sort of resemble (except maybe a little pointier) when their chaff or husk has been removed. Otherwise they're a pretty red color. The plant is actually a little hardier than regular old wheat, which is usually a hybrid of some kind. Spelt was first grown in the US around the turn of the century. Nowadays it's fed mostly to farm animals, which is too bad, because it's healthy for humans, containing about 12% protein (about as much as oats) and a good share of fiber, calcium, and iron. To prepare the stuff, combine about 4 cups of water and 1-1/4 cups spelt, bring it all to a boil, then cook gently for about an hour. It can be eaten as a cereal for breakfast, or with vegetables and things. It doesn't have much gluten, but it can be used to make a dense bread, as follows:

Mix together 3-1/2 cups spelt flour (you can buy berries and grind them yourself if you'd like), 2 tbsp. baking soda, 1 teaspoon of sea salt, 1-1/2 cups of water, and 1/2 cup of apple butter or organic applesauce for sweetening. Pour the batter into an oiled pan and bake for about 40 minutes at 350∞.

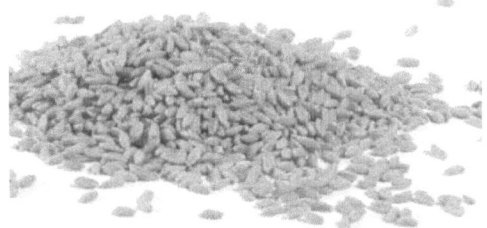

http://www.ncwheatmontanacoop.com

SPIRULINA

is a blue-green algae that grows in a twisty, spiral sort of shape. It's been around on the planet for about 3.6 billion years, but has only recently gotten popular as a super-nutritious and earth-friendly food. A company called "Earthrise," who started growing it in California in 1982, says it's "earth's healthiest food," and that it yields more nutrition per acre than any known plant and absorbs more carbon dioxide (and makes more oxygen) than even a rain forest. It's 3.5 times more energy-efficient (input vs. output) to produce than even soybeans (not to mention over 100 times more than beef), and uses 1/3 of the water (8 gallons per serving vs. 136 gallons for an egg and 1,300 for a burger). This micro-algae even kicks soy's butt in the nutrition arena, with 20 times more protein (at 65%, it's the champion of the plant world). Better yet, its cell walls are made mostly of protein, so it's easier for the body to use it (most other plant cell walls are mostly cellulose, which has to be broken down). It's also the world's best source of vitamin B12 (it's got twice as much as liver), iron, calcium, and magnesium, and has a good supply of essential fatty acids, including GLA, being the only whole food besides mother's milk with this rare ingredient. Spirulina is also the best place to get beta carotene, a nutrient that does wonders for the immune system. In fact, the little plant was patented in Russia as a treatment for radiation sickness after it helped Chernobyl survivors, and seems to help AIDS patients, too. To top it all off, the chlorophyll in spirulina will help clean out your liver, kidneys, and arteries, and generally enrich your blood. It's a natural appetite suppressant, offers pure glycogen (which gives the body energy) and may even slow down aging. Spirulina is sold in tablets (to be taken like vitamins), or as a powder, one teaspoon of which can be added to juice, soup, or water to get a good daily supply of health.

SPROUTS

When seeds, beans, or grains germinate, they become full of life and packed with vitamins and nutrients for the little plant to grow big and strong. In fact, within a few days, the content of vitamins A, B, and E increases up to 300%, depending on the type of seed, and vitamin C, which is usually lacking, increases up to 700% and gives sprouts as much as (or, in some seeds, up to 6 times more than) the same amount of citrus. All these vitamins (and the plentiful enzymes that come along with them) also help humans get (or stay) big and strong, and help detoxify the body. Sprouts also contain all the essential aminos and fatty acids, lots of calcium, iron, and chlorophyll (see wheatgrass juice). What few calories they do have are in the form of simple plant sugars that provide quick energy. Given the right amount of moisture and air (lots), light (minimal, especially at first), and the right temperature (75-80 degrees), sprouts can be grown quickly (in less than a week) and cheaply (4 oz. of seeds yields about a pound) at any time of year. If rinsed with cool water every now and then, they can be stored in the fridge for a week or more. Among the things good for sprouting are alfalfa, buckwheat, lentils, mung beans, radish, red clover, and sunflower. It's best to use seeds that have been grown especially for sprouting and to avoid anything treated with chemicals or dyes. Each variety has a different taste and texture, but they're all chock full of goodness. Eat some on a sandwich or in (or as) a salad.

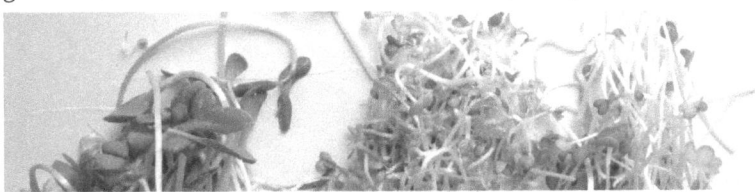

http://www.seasonalchef.com

STEVIA

(S. *rebaudiana*) is an evergreen shrub from the northern part of South America whose leaves have been used since ancient times to sweeten things like the herbal tea and "mate" that people in Brazil and Paraguay have been known to drink. It is said to be thirty times sweeter than refined sugar, has no calories, and, unlike most sweeteners that just sweeten, it might even be good for you. Plus, it can be used by those with hypoglycemia and diabetes. The first white folks to find out about stevia (or *Ka he'e* as the natives call it) were the Conquistadors, who spread the word to Spain. Early in this century, a guy named Dr. Bertoni told people in America, while in other places like Korea and Japan, a natural extraction called stevioside has been used since the '70s to sweeten diet Coke, soy sauce, and other goodies. In 1987, the company that makes Nutrasweet heard about stevia and complained to the FDA, who suddenly started calling it an "unapproved food additive" (even though it's not really an additive, but an actual food), and told people they had to stop using and selling it until it went through all kinds of expensive testing (Nutrasweet, by the way, has been tested and linked to various unpleasantries like blindness and brain tumors). Thanks to the American Herbal Products Association, though, who made a good case for its safety, stevia isn't illegal anymore, although it still can't officially be labeled as a "sweetener" until The Man says it's alright.

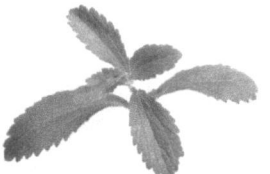

http://blog.zevia.com

SUCANAT,

a word made from the first part of the words sugar cane natural, is a sweetener made from the juice of organic sugar cane. The cane is pressed, and its liquid is then co-crystallized with a little molasses, resulting in a light brown substance that's tastier and far less processed than white sugar. It's also healthier, as it retains some of the cane's minerals (especially calcium, potassium, and magnesium) and trace vitamins (like A and C), while refined sugar is 99.9% sucrose and 0% nutrition. At 80-90% sucrose, Sucanat produces a lower glycemic response, which means it may be safe for some diabetics, depending on one's metabolism. Sucanat is sometimes called "evaporated cane juice," although this officially refers to a lighter version made without molasses. It's also called Florida Crystals, although it's actually made up of little, round granules which dissolve instantly in water and blend more thoroughly with other ingredients than sugar crystals. Sucanat, which also comes in a powdered form, has a long shelf life. It can be substituted 1:1 in place of white sugar, brown sugar, and honey, in cookies, cakes, and other yummies.

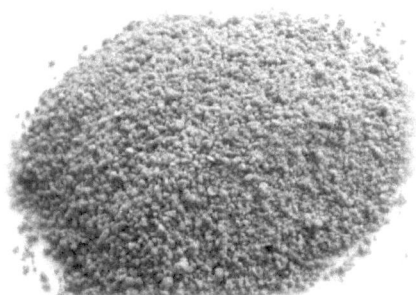

http://www.purcellmountainfarms.com

SUMA

Indigenous to the tropics of Central and South America, this shrubby ground vine is sometimes called "Brazilian ginseng," though it's not actually from the *Panax* family but from the Amaranth family. Like ginseng, however, the roots of *Pfaffia panicula* have for ages been considered a general energy and health rejuvenator. In fact, suma is known down south as "para toda" ("for all things"), as it's been employed to improve and regulate the cardiovascular and nervous systems, digestion, hormonal secretions, immunity, and sexual functions. In America and Europe, it's gotten popular as a treatment for chronic fatigue, arthritis, diabetes, high cholesterol and blood pressure, even leukemia and cancer. Russian Olympic athletes have been known to consume suma instead of steroids, earning it the nickname "The Russian Secret." It was in Russia, by the way, that N.V. Lazarev coined the term "adaptogen" in 1947 to describe substances which "increase the body's resistance to adverse influences by a wide range of biochemical reactions," which suma certainly does. Apart from containing a good dose of amino acids and familiar nutrients like vitamins A, B1, B2, E, and pantothenic acid, suma is also a good source of the obscure trace element germanium, which supposedly helps oxygenate cells, as well as being a storehouse of saponins including certain "pfaffosides" and "pfaffic acids" that inhibit the growth of tumors (scientists in both Japan and America have patented synthetic versions of these). Another of suma's weird ingredients, called beta ecdysterene, works on the immune system and may be responsible for the steroid-like effects that gave the Russians their edge. Dried suma root is hard to come by, but a powdered form is available in pills.

SWEET POTATO

Often spelled as one word these days, this member of the morning glory family originated in tropical Central or South America. Clues suggest that it may have been cultivated as early as 8,000 BCE (making it one of the first domesticated plants), though it was certainly widespread in the Americas by 4500 BCE Early Spanish explorers brought the sweetpotato back to Europe, while the Portugese introduced it to Africa, India, and Asia. In Polynesia, "uala" used to be a staple whose cultivation was shared by both men and women. The sweetpotato is now about the 7th most economically important crop in the world, and, being drought-resistant *and* nutritious (see below), it's *the* most important root crop in developing regions, where almost 95% of sweetpotatoes are grown (the country that consumes the most is China). In some places, the leaves of *Ipomoea batata* are eaten as greens, but the famous part is obviously the underground part, known as a "storage root" rather than a "tuber," which is actually a modified stem. This vegetable has loads of potassium, calcium, iron, thiamine (B1), and Vitamin C, while the orange-fleshed variety packs about twice the RDA of Vitamin A. Sweetpotatoes can be cooked and mashed in a million ways, but they retain the most nutrition when baked and eaten with the skin. Although the words "sweetpotato" and "yam" are used interchaneably in the US, the yam is a different species with its roots in Africa (its name comes from the West African word "nyami"). Generally, yams are more rough and scaly outside, less moist and sweet inside.

TAHINI, SESAME BUTTER, AND SESAME SALT

are different things, but they all come from the same sesame plant, which is native to India. People around those parts regard sesame as a symbol of immortality. It's one of the oldest sources of oil and spice (and lots of things nice), but until the invention of a non-scattering variety, it was hard to cultivate the seeds because of their tendency to fall off and blow away when they got ripe. **Tahini** is a paste made from ground, hulled, unroasted seeds. It's popular in the Middle East, where people put it in things like halva and hummus, which is made with chick peas. **Sesame butter**, on the other hand, is ground from roasted, unhulled seeds, and is therefore darker and a little better for you. Both concoctions, however, are high in protein, iron, calcium, vitamins and minerals, and are tasty, too. They can be used in salad dressings and sauces, added to soups or cooking rice to add a nutty flavor, or spread right on bread and rice cakes. Gomaiso, or **sesame salt**, can me made by grinding together (by hand, preferably) about 20 teaspoons of seeds and a teaspoon of salt. Sprinkle this condiment on rice or veggies or oatmeal. It's said to help headaches and to calm crybabies.

The Japanese character for tamari has been found in documents dated as early as 776 BCE. It means "soybean filtering," as it referred to the dark liquid that rose to the surface during the fermentation of miso. This salty solution became popular as a seasoning sauce known as tamari-shoyu, made from water, salt, soybeans, and roasted barley. Eventually, wheat was used instead of barley, and the result, called "shoyu," was later enjoyed by the likes of Louis XIV. Traditionally, shoyu was allowed to age for years in cedar vats, but its modern ancestor, soy sauce, is usually made quickly and synthetically with added junk like corn syrup, MSG, preservatives, even hydrochloric acid. Fortunately, what's nowadays sold as "tamari" is brewed the old-fashioned way. It's used to flavor soups, rice, noodles, veggies, sauces and broths, or for sautéeing and basting, and mixes well with other condiments. Combine it with lemon juice and wasabi to make a tangy dip.

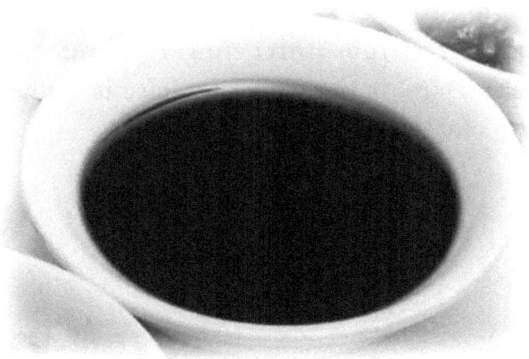

http://www.enlightenedcooking.blogspot.com

135

TARO

The earliest official mention of this plant, a.k.a. "malanga," was in 23 BCE by Greeks who found it growing in Egypt, although it most likely came from India or Southeast Asia. For ages it's been an important food for Caribbeans, Polynesians, and also West Africans, who probably brought it to America on slave ships. These days, most American "dasheen" is grown in Florida, where it was first introduced as a substitute for potatoes, which don't do as well in the wet soil down there. In the Caribbean, taro's large leaves, or "callaloo," are eaten raw like mustard greens, but in some varieties they have to be cooked first to get rid of a toxin called calcium oxalate. In other types, such as Chinese taro, the stems are also edible. Taro's most famous part, though, is by far the root or chubby, underground stem called the "corm." This tuber, brown outside and grayish or even purply inside, has lots of calcium, iron, phosphorus, and vitamin B, and almost no fat. Its tiny starch grains make it easy for even the weakest stomachs to digest. In fact, in Hawaii, where the "kalo" plant is sacred, there is no word for "indigestion." On those islands, the root is often ground, combined with water, and fermented to make "poi." This sour paste is eaten with the hands and ranges from "three-finger" (thin) to "one-finger" (thick). Here on the mainland, taro is sometimes seen in the form of chips.

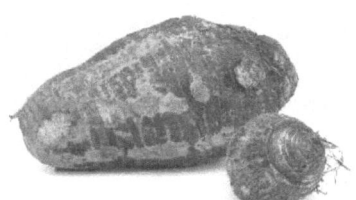

http://www.foodsubs.com

TEA TREE OIL

When explorer Captain James Cook came to Australia in the 1770s, he noticed that the indigenous folks often chewed the leaves of a certain relative of eucalytus to treat illness, and also used the leaves to make a tea, which inspired the tree's popular name. Nowadays, the fast-growing foliage of *Melaleuca alterifolia* is harvested from plantations by machine, and its camphorous essential oil is steam-distilled and added to soaps, deodorants, toothpastes, lotions, lozenges and cleaning products. The oil itself is one of the strongest known natural germ-fighters, with additional power to combat viruses, fungi, and at least 11 types of bacteria. When applied to the skin, it rejuvenates the cells and helps heal cuts, burns, bug bites, bee stings, rashes, boils, pimples, and canker sores. It eliminates dandruff, ringworm and lice on the head, sore throat in the gullet, athlete's foot on the feet, and yeast infection. Tea tree oil is one of the few essential oils that is rich enough to be used alone (without being added to a heavier base oil) and has been shown to have effects that last days and even weeks after application.

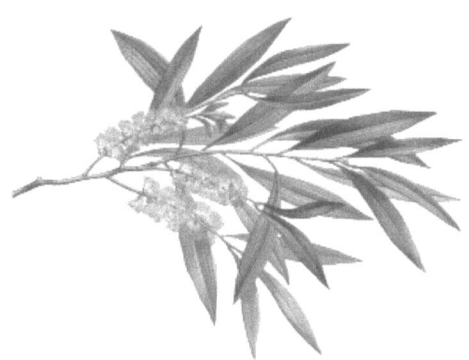

http://www.wondersoftea.com

137

TEFF

is a type of Ethiopian wild grass grown for its grain, which is the littlest in the world — smaller, in fact, than the dot over the "i" in "tiny," and weighing less than 1/100th as much as a grain of wheat. Its name actually means "lost," as in: if you drop a grain of it, you can kiss the little feller goodbye. In addition to being wee, teff is pretty darn ancient. Its seeds have been found in bricks used to build pyramids in Egypt. These days, Ethiopians use its straw to make adobe dwellings (for people who aren't so royal or dead), and its flour to make a traditional flatbread. It's also grown in Australia, Europe, and Idaho. Fortunately, teff is too small to hull, so it gets to keep its nutrition-packed bran and germ, which it has more of (relative to its size) than any other grain. Gram for gram, it has 17 times the calcium of whole wheat or barley, and is high in protein, iron, and complex carbos. Teff makes a good, gluten-free flapjack or quickbread batter, and can be boiled into a porridge.

To make Ethiopian injeras: mix 2 cups of teff flour with 2.5 cups of lukewarm water, and let ferment for 2 or 3 days. This mixture is sometimes combined with a batter made from the same amounts of a rising flour (like wheat or barley) and water, and 1/2 tsp baking soda. If using this method, let the resulting mixture sit a couple hours before frying, which is done in a big skillet. Pour the batter a little thicker than a crépe, and wait for it to bubble. Injeras are used as edible plates and edible utensils with which to scoop food.

TEMPEH

(pronounced "TEM-pay") is an Indonesian soyfood which, unlike tofu, contains whole beans (and sometimes other grains) which are held together by a stringy type of bacteria. Though it sounds a little gross, this mycelium is high in fiber and B vitamins (uncluding B12), and makes the beans, which contribute to tempeh's 20% protein content, easy to digest. Tempeh's flavor has been described as "nutty," "yeasty" and "mushroomy," but it also readily absorbs marinades and seasonings. It can be baked, broiled, boiled, steamed, or fried and added to soups, combined with vegetables, or ground into spreads.

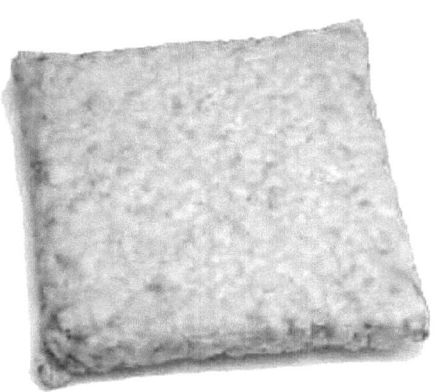

http://www.foodsubs.com

TEXTURED SOY PROTEIN

TSP is made from compressed soy flour, which in turn is made from roasted, ground soybeans. It looks and tastes a lot like "textured vegetable protein," made from dehydrated, defatted beans, although TVP is a registered trademark of Archer Daniels Midland Company, who uses it in their "Harvest Burgers," a top-selling American soy product. "Soya texturizado" is also popular in Mexico, where it's three times cheaper than meat, and a heck of a lot healthier. It contains no cholesterol, hardly any fat or sodium, lots of protein (up to 70%, depending on how it's processed), fiber, and minerals like zinc. It is sold granulated, flaked, or in larger chunks, all of which need to be rehydrated by adding an equal amount of boiling water. After sitting for 25 minutes or so, the TSP will have the texture of ground beef, and can be used in sloppy joes (or joans), tacos, chili, spaghetti sauce, and other traditionally meaty dishes. Texturized vegetable protein is not to be confused with hydrolized vegetable protein (HVP), protein that has been extracted from any vegetable and broken down into amino acids, usually used in soup stocks or as a flavor enhancer.

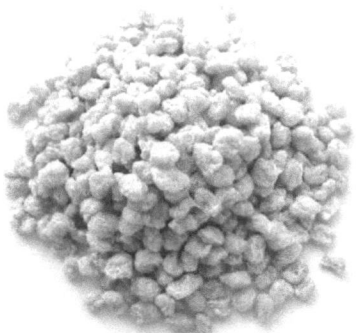

http://www.made-in-china.com

THYME

Use of this herb goes way back to ancient Egypt, when it was a part of mummy-making, and ancient Greece, where it was burned to ward off disease and insects. Folks in Scotland, who believed the low, bushy perennial to be the home of fairies, consumed the stuff to prevent scary dreams and increase bravery. The genus *Thymus*, which, in fact, means "courage," contains at least 50 species, the most famous being *T. vulgaris*, or common thyme, and *T. serpyllium*, or Mother-of-thyme. Both of these are grown mainly for decoration, while Narrow-Leaf French, Broadleaf English, and Lemon Thyme are the most common culinary varieties. In all types, the leaves and little flowers are the parts that get eaten, whether contributing their somewhat minty flavor to soups, salads, and such, or helping to cure coughs, colds, congestion, and tummy ailments. Sometimes thyme tea is gargled to relieve a sore throat, or drunk with fenugreek to clear the lungs, and at one time, thyme oil (or "thymol") was a popular antiseptic. Nutritionally, thyme is full of vitamins C, D, and the Bs (especially thiamine), and trace minerals. When cooking, use about three times as much fresh thyme as dried, although in either case you'll rarely need more than a pinch.

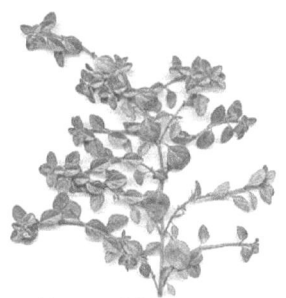

http://www.sfakia-crete.com

TOMATOES

A member of the nightshade family, the tomato plant was first domesticated in South America by the Incas. Its fruit was originally rough and ridged, until a European gardener began breeding the smooth, round "Paragon" type that's now the most widely grown "vegetable" in the US (although, as the reproductive structure of a flowering plant, it's technically a fruit, which you probably already knew). Anyway, the "love apple," as it was called last century, gets its ruddy color from "lycopene," a pigment found in lesser quantities in watermelon, guava, and pink grapefruit. Lycopene has recently been shown by folks at Harvard Medical School to reduce the risk of certain cancers (especially those of the prostate, lung, and stomach) up to 34% in subjects who ate 2 or more servings of tomato-based foodstuffs per week (versus none). As it turns out, lycopene is also the most powerful antioxidant in the family of carotenoids, which includes beta carotene (provitamin A) and alpha carotene (the color in carrots). As such, it freely donates its electrons to unstable oxygen molecules (free rads), helping to repair damage done by ultraviolet radiation (such as sunburn) as well as preventing bad cholesterol from being converted into artery-clogging plaque, thereby reducing the risk of heart attack (by as much as 50% in one study). Lycopene seems to be most abundant in cooked tomato products, such as tomato sauce, tomato juice, and ketchup. Its "bioavailability" is especially high in tomato paste, which has twice the lycopene concentration of raw tomatoes and 4 times the rate of absorption into the bloodstream.

said to be the first truly human-made cereal, is a cross between wheat and rye. These two grains, which have a common ancestor, have been cross-bred for about a hundred years, but it wasn't until the 1930s that the first fertile hybrids showed up. Triticale combines the goodness of both of its parents, and is even better in some ways. It has a higher yield per acre than either crop (which means more food and less reliance on pesticides and junk), and seems to grow good in bad soil and cold weather. It has at least as much protein (10-13%) and amino acids as its parents, and 40% more fiber than wheat. Fiber is good for the guts, and helps prevent heart disease, diabetes, and cancer, especially the kind that strikes the colon (I'm not talking punctuation marks). Unfortunately, most triticale is eaten by farm animals. The grains of this plant are bigger than wheat or rye. They have an aromatic smell and a naturally sweet, delicious taste. Use them in soups, breakfast porridges, and other recipes that call for wheat. To make bread, mix in a little wheat flour to get the gluten that's lacking in this new-fangled food.

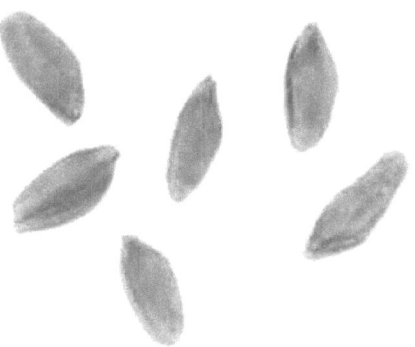

http://www.foodsubs.com

TURMERIC

Also spelled "tumeric," this spice comes from the dried, ground roots of *Curcuma longa*, a relative of ginger that's native to India and southeast Asia. The plant's genus name is derived from "kirkum," a Persian word meaning "saffron," which turmeric resembles in its bright orange, powdered form. On a trip to China in 1280, Marco Polo himself wrote about a plant with the qualities of saffron that wasn't saffron, and Medieval Europeans called the spice "Indian saffron." Not just a cheap substitute for a pricey spice, turmeric has been used for millennia in Ayurvedic medicine to treat coughs and poor vision, boost the immune system, purify the blood, limber up the ligaments before yoga, and impart the energy of the Divine Mother. It has value in traditional Chinese medicine and on certain islands in the Pacific, where it was sprinkled on the shoulders during religious rituals. Throughout the world and the ages, turmeric has also been used to treat acne, arthritis, allergies, burns, digestive and liver disorders, and ulcers; to make perfumes and soaps, to preserve food, and to dye cloth. Turmeric's most common job these days is lending its color to yellow mustard and to curry powder, a mixture of spices which might include coriander, fenugreek, pepper, cumin, cardamom, cloves, and chili. Modern scientists have isolated the active ingredient in turmeric as "curcumin," and have shown that it acts as an antioxidant at least as powerful as Vitamin E, neutralizes carcinogens and inhibits tumor growth, relieves congestion and inflammation, works like aspirin to kill pain, and has antiseptic, antibacterial, and antiviral properties. Usually sold in its colorful powdered form, turmeric also comes in tablets and in an oil commonly used to color stuff.

UMEBOSHI PLUMS

The plant from which this sour plum comes is actually native to China, but it has become more popular in Japan. Its fruit is picked and pickled with salt to produce umeboshi vinegar, which serves as a sharp addition to dressings or sweet-and-sour sauces. The plums, though originally green, turn red due to contact with "shiso" leaves, with which they are pickled, and also become saltier and more alkaline. For this reason, they are often eaten to neutralize acidity in the blood and to help digestion.

To make a dressing, add some plum slices (or plum vinegar) to apple juice, sesame oil, and tamari.

For a hot cold remedy, add a plum to 1 1/2 pints of water, 1/2 tsp. grated ginger, and a teaspoon of kuzu. Boil until the liquid is transparent and drink while hot.

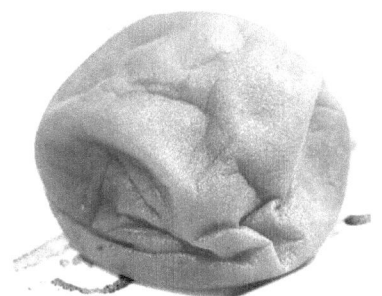

http://a-eda.net

WASABI

is a spicy Japanese horseradish with a pale green color and a pungent taste. It's usually eaten with sushi as a condiment (often mixed with tamari or soy sauce to make a dip), and can be used to liven up any soup, sauce, or noodle salad. Wasabi is sold either as a paste or a powder, the latter needing to be mixed with water, stirred, and set aside for awhile before use. A little wasabi goes a long way, as it's quite tangy. Interestingly, however, its spicyness doesn't linger in the mouth, but rises, in a short but intense rush, from the tongue through the nasal passages and seemingly out the eyes.

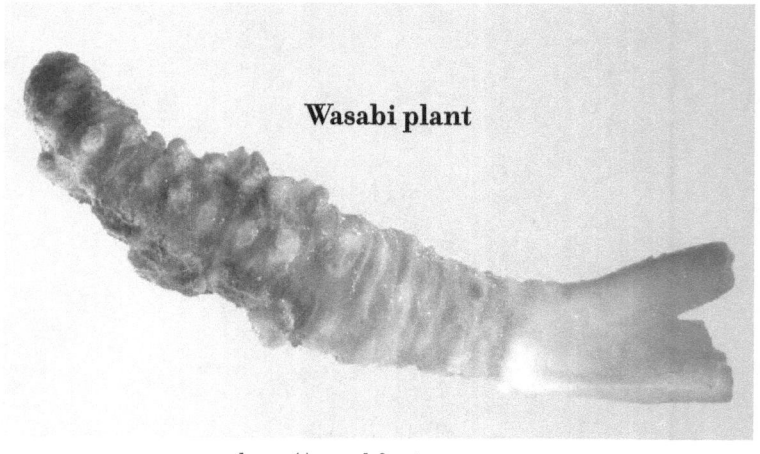

Wasabi plant

http://www.kfunigraz.ac.at

WHEAT GERM

Wheat has been the "staff of life" since forever, starting in Mesopotamia and Egypt, then spreading from Rome into Europe. Columbus brought some on his little voyage in 1492, and Cortez took the stuff to Mexico in 1519. It's now the most popular cereal grain, maybe because it has a goodly amount of gluten needed to make decent bread. There are over 30,000 varieties of *triticum*, the three most famous being the high-protein "hard wheat," the lower-protein "soft wheat," and "durham" wheat, which is usually ground to make semolina flour for pasta. The grain itself, also called the kernel or berry, is composed of 14.5% bran (the outer layer), 83% endosperm (the part usually ground into flour), and 2.5% germ, the embryo of the new plant. The germ is the kernel's nutritional heart, containing 30% protein, lots of B vitamins (especially B2, B3, and B6), and minerals like iron, manganese and copper. It's also pretty fatty, and for this reason wheat germ is often toasted to extend its short shelf life. In this form, it can be added to flours or even soups and smoothies in order to boost protein content. Wheat germ is sometimes pressed into a strongly-flavored oil, and is also available as a powdered extract. Another place to find it is in whole wheat flour, which also retains the high-fiber bran that otherwise gets milled right off.

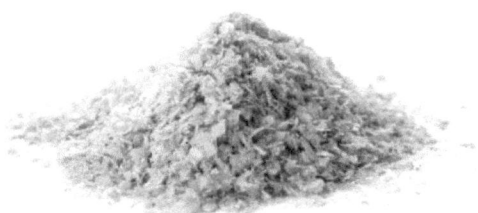

http://www.thedailygreen.com

WHEATGRASS JUICE

Wheatgrass is sprouted from wheat berries, usually the red variety, which makes the most nutritious little plantlings. The grass itself is the most full of nutrition when about eight inches tall, but it's also full of cellulose and other fibers that human stomachs can't digest, so it has to be juiced and strained. In this form, it has all the B and E vitamins, complete proteins, and enzymes that all sprouts have, is an even better source for vitamins A and C, and may be the very best place to get calcium, iron, magnesium, and potassium. One ounce of the stuff has about the same nutritional value as 2 1/2 lbs. of green, leafy veggies. Perhaps the best thing about wheatgrass juice is its amazing 70% chlorophyll content (which contributes to its "planty" taste). Chlorophyll is sometimes called "green blood" because it matches the structure of hemoglobin except for having an atom of magnesium instead of iron in the middle. It cleans and builds the blood and cells, and fights bacteria, especially the kinds that cause B.O. When given a gargle, wheatgrass juice freshens the breath while nutrifying the gums, or will soothe a sore throat. In the shnoz, it will relieve congestion and inflamed sinuses. It's good for the scalp, and is said to keep away gray hair, if you're scared of that kind of thing. Its enzymes have even been linked to cures for cancer. The best way to get the goodness from wheatgrass is to juice it yourself and drink it right away, but the juicing contraptions are kind of expensive. It's available frozen (to be blended into juices), or freeze-dried into a powder, which actually boosts its protein content up to 48% (3 times that of beef).

WILD CELERY SEEDS

From the same family as carrots and parsley comes the 2- to 3-foot tall *Apium graveolens*, commonly called "smallage." Although modern humans favor the crunchy stalk of its domesticated ancestor, the wild variety has been prized throughout the ages for its tiny, brown fruits (or so-called seeds), about 75,000 of which weigh one pound. People of the Mediterranean region (the plant's place of origin) have used wild celery seeds to flavor food since the time of the ancient Greeks, who also used the plant's leaves to honor winners of sporting events (ancient Romans, on the other hand, employed the foliage to decorate coffins). The early European herbalist Nicholas Culpepper, who associated smallage with Mercury, noted its effect on arthritis, rheumatism, gout, "foul ulcers and cankers," as well as its ability "to help a stinking breath." In Ayurvedic medicine, wild celery seeds, or *ajwan*, are considered useful for clearing away *ama* or toxic buildup, especially in the digestive and respiratory tracts, and for vitalizing the energy governing effort, enthusiasm, and aspiration. Recent studies have shown these seeds to be effective against high blood pressure and cholesterol, while one study at the University of Minnesota found that they reduce the incidence of tumors (in mice) by as much as 57%, possibly due to the chemicals sedanolide and (butyl) phthaladide. Besides these fancy ingredients, wild celery seeds also contain potassium and good old Vitamin C. Grown commercially in places like France and India, the seeds are harvested, dried, and then often crushed, either to be infused to make tea, or combined with fine table salt to make the popular spice and condiment known as celery salt.

WILD RICE

isn't actually rice, but the seeds of *Zizania aquatica*, a plant that grows in marshes in Minnesota, where it's the state grain. The Chippewa (or Ojibwa) call it "mahnoomin" (which means "good berry") and have been harvesting it for over 800 years. Traditional "ricing" happens in September and involves canoeing through the 10' tall reeds, bending them down with a piece of wood, and tapping the ripe seeds loose with another, "knocker" stick. The green seeds are dried and parched over a fire, then hulled (back in the day, this was done by foot). In the early '60s, white people figured out how to grow "wild" rice in artificial paddies and harvest it by machine. When seen in the store, these grains look black (because of the drying method) and shiny (because of the processing), instead of matte brown, light brown and green, like the organic kind. Nutritionally, mahnoomin beats cultivated cereals (like wheat oats, rye, and barley) grains down. It's got about 14% protein, lots of potassium, phosphorus, and B vitamins (especially niacin), loads of carbos for energy, and almost no fat. To prepare it, use 4 cups water to 1 cup rice, and boil for about 20 minutes. The processed variety takes about twice as long to cook. Wild rice is good in soups and stuffing, and goes well with dried fruit and nuts to make a pilaf.

http://www.gourmetsleuth.com

WINGED BEANS

The plant from which these legumes come is native to New Guinea, but is now being cultivated in other tropical areas because of its sustainability and nutritional goodness. This "food of the future" grows fast, resists disease, and raises the fertility of the soil by fixing the nitrogen content. Best yet, the entire plant, from the roots to the spinachy leaves to the colorful flowers, is edible. The tuber weighs in at around 30% carbohydrates and 15-20% protein, and is eaten either raw or cooked. The pods, ranging in color from green to purple or red, flare at one end into four "wings" (thus the name). If picked when young, they cook up and taste kind of like green beans. The seeds/beans themselves contain an impressive 30-40% protein, some of it in the form of "lectins," chemicals that help the immune system. They also contain erucic acid, often used as an anti-tumor medication. Also called goa or princess beans, they are similar in composition to soybeans, and can be processed into tofu and tempeh, or liquified into a tasty beverage.

http://www.geocities.jp

YACON

(pronounced ya-cone), refers mainly to an alternative sweetener made from the tuberous roots of *Smallanthus sonchifolius*, which is indigenous to the Andes mountains. The plant was used by the ancient Incas, and the tuber is still eaten by Bolivians and Peruvians as a fruit-like vegetable with a flavor and texture somewhere between apples and celery. Yacon tubers, which become even sweeter when dried, have the remarkable quality of being low in calories and glucose levels; lower, in fact, than any other sweetener apart from stevia. Yacon instead contains a form of fructose called inulin, which is difficult for the body to break down and also promotes the growth of beneficial bacteria in the gut. Since yacon doesn't raise blood sugar levels, it's an ideal sweetener for diabetics and weight-watchers, while everyone can benefit from its antioxidants, minerals, and yummy caramel taste.

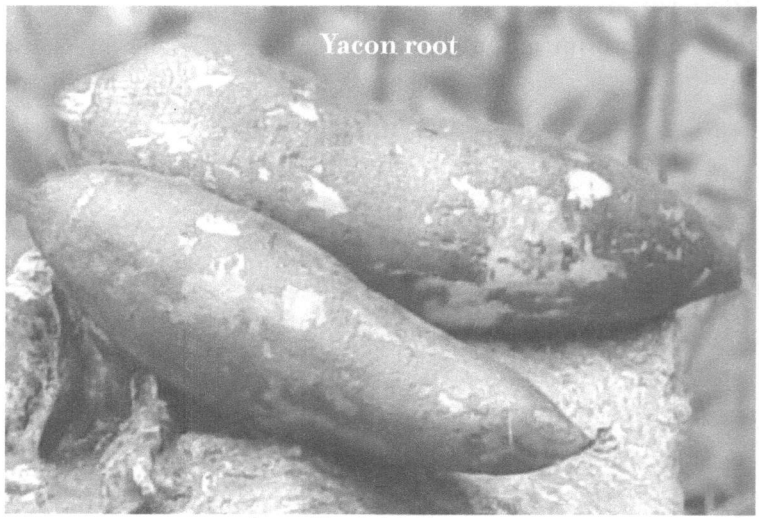

Yacon root

http://herbalguides.com

YAMABUSHITAKE

The various common names for this medicinal mushroom – which include "Monkey's Head," "Lion's Mane," "Hedgehog fungus," and "Beard fungus" – all provide some description of its striking appearance. Germinating on fallen logs, stumps, and wounded parts of live trees in Asia, Europe, and parts of North America, *Hericium erinaceus* grows as a roundish cluster of drooping, off-white tendrils or tufts. As one of the "8 most precious gourmets" in China, so-called "Hou Tou Gu" has been used in Traditional Chinese Medicine to benefit the stomach and spleen as well as strengthen the body as a whole. Recent scientific evidence suggests that yamabushitake may lower cholesterol and high blood pressure as well as boost immunity, while the polysaccharides it contains may inhibit the RNA and DNA in cancer cells, preventing their growth and reproduction. Rich in protein, this functional fungal food also contains a compound called "Nerve Growth Stimulant Factor," which nurtures neurons and may help curb Alzheimer's, senility, and even enhance intelligence. The flavor of yamabushitake is said to be similar to that of lobster of crab, for which it sometimes serves as a substitute in salads and stir-fries. If picked while young, the tendrils tend to be slightly rubbery, while more mature mushrooms are yellowed and sour-tasting.

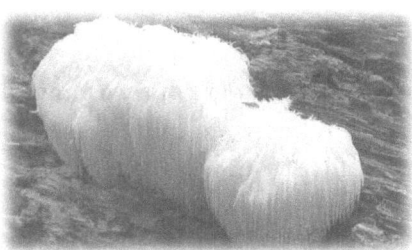

http://www.sierrapotomac.org

153

YARROW

Fossilized pollen grains from this member of the Sunflower family suggest that it may have been used as much as 50,000 years ago by Neanderthals. Certainly *Homo sapiens* has known about *Achillea millefolium* since ancient Greece, when *herba militaris* (the military herb) was used to stop the bleeding of wounded soldiers, perhaps by Achilles himself (hence the plant's genus name). Yarrow's hemostatic action has led to the names "Bloodwort" and "Nosebleed." The herb also goes by "Lady's Mantle," "All-Heal," "Milfoil," and "Thousand Leaf," the last two referring to the species name and the plant's abundance of little leaves, whose peppery taste has landed them in salads and snuff (hence another label, "Old Man's Pepper"). Yarrow has finally been called "Devil's Nettle" because of its use in divination methods, such as the tossing of dried yarrow stalks before consulting the *I Ching*, and the tickling of the inside of the nose with a yarrow leaf to see if it bleeds favorably. Despite all this flap about its leaves, yarrow's main medicinal component is its delicate, whitish or pinkish flowers and upper stems, which, when consumed as a tea, help eliminate toxins, partly by making a person sweat, thereby warding off oncoming colds and flu. Yarrow is also good for inflammation, congestion, tooth and gum aches, and high blood pressure. It can help with things like hemmorhoids, scrapes, and rashes, but in the event of serious bleeding, it would be a good idea to go to the hospital if there's one around. Yarrow is not recommended for pregant moms, and has been known to cause some side effects, such as sensitivity to sunlight, after long-term use.

refers to a beverage made from *Ilex paraguayensis*, a bushy, South American evergreen tree related to holly. Ages ago, Guarani Indians in Paraguay drank this "gourd tea" to boost immunity and ward off fatigue and hunger, as did *gouchos* (Argentinian cowboys) later on. Thanks to Jesuit priests, the drink was commercialized in the 1600s, and it's still big business in Brazil and Argentina, where it's the national pick-me-up. In Paraguay, it's still harvested from the wild, which helps preserve the forests and the livelihood of indigenous forest-dwelling peoples. The traditional method of consuming mate (pronounced MAH tay), still practiced in most of South America, involves putting some dried, crushed leaves into a calabasa gourd (or a cup made of wood, cow horn, silver, or porcelain-covered steel), letting them steep in hot water, then drinking the tea through a tube called a "bombilla," which has a strainer on one end and a heat-resistant, gold tip at the other. Of course, if you don't have a gourd and a fancy straw, you can just strain the tea after steeping. Plant parts other than the leaves can also be used, and other herbs can be thrown in to make a milder, less bitter concoction. The magical stimulant in yerba mate is called mateine, a "xanthinoid" similar to caffeine, but without its addictive properties or jittery side effects. Mateine is said to produce a much "cleaner," longer-lasting buzz, and can actually improve the quality of your sleep rather than cause insomnia. It relaxes smooth muscles and improves blood flow, aids digestion and (ahem) evacuation and may even help regenerate cells. On top of it all, yerba mate contains ample quantities of vitamins B1, B2, and C, plus minerals like iron, calcium, phosphorus, and managnese. This has led some people to call it "Nature's most perfect beverage" and even "beverage of the gods," but that's getting a little carried away.

are vitamins, minerals, enzymes, or plant pigments that protect the body from toxic buildup by attacking unstable oxygen molecules in the body. In addition to defending against these "free radicals," antioxidants also nourish and strengthen the immune system. See GRAPESEEDS for another antioxidant synopsis. The following pages provide information on the most common antioxidants and list featured foodstuffs in which they can be found.

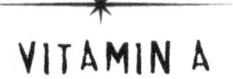

VITAMIN A

One of the strongest antioxidants, this vitamin gets stored in the liver and fatty tisue, which is where most toxins hang out. It maintains healthy epithelial tissue in the skin, lungs, and mucous membranes, where over half of all cancers occur. Vitamin A also protects the skin from harmful ultraviolet radiation, and is needed for good eyesight. Plant foods, interestingly, do not contain this vitamin, but do contain beta carotene, which gets quickly coverted by the body into vitamin A. American diets tend to be lacking in this important antioxidant. Sources include ALOE VERA JUICE, ASPARAGUS, ARAME, BOK CHOY, CHLORELLA, DONG QUAI, DUNALLIELLA, FAVA BEANS, FENNEL, FIDDLEHEAD FERNS, GARLIC, GOJI BERRIES, GOTU KOLA, HEMP SEEDS, KALE, MAITAKE, OKRA, OREGANO, PARSLEY, PUMPKIN, RAPINI, ROOIBOS, ROYAL JELLY, SAGE, SARSAPARILLA, SORREL, SPIRULINA, SUMA, SWETPOTATO, and WHEATGRASS JUICE.

B COMPLEX

Some common members of this team are B1 (thiamine), B2

(riboflavin), B3 (niacin), B5 (pantothenic acid), B6 (pyri-
doxine), B12 (cobalamin), folic acid, choline, and PABA.
These vitamins help the body make antibodies and metabo-
lize proteins and fats, boost energy and regulate the liver
and kidneys. They are also related to mental health and the
nerves. The elusive B12 can be found in ALOE VERA JUICE,
BARLEY GRASS, CHLORELLA, DONG QUAI, GOJI BERRIES,
MACA, MISO, NATTO, TEMPEH, AND SPIRULINA; other
types come in ARAME, ALFALFA, ALOE VERA JUICE,
ASPARAGUS, BOK CHOY, BREWER'S YEAST, BROWN RICE,
FAVA BEANS, GARLIC, GOJI BERRIES, GOTU KOLA, HEMP
SEEDS, KAMUT, LENTILS, MACA, MAITAKE, MOLASSES,
NATTO, OKRA, PARSLEY, ROYAL JELLY, SEITAN, SHII-
TAKE, SPROUTS, SUMA, SWEETPOTATO, WHEATGRASS
JUICE, WILD RICE and YERBA MATE.

VITAMIN C.

also called "ascorbic acid," neutralizes over 50 known toxins,
boosts the immune system and helps the body process iron.
Being similar in composition to sugar, it can be sythesized
from glucose by most animals except monkeys, guinea pigs,
Indian fruit bats, and humans. It is the least stable vitamin,
sensitive to heat, light, and air, and is eliminated from the body
within a few hours. Its absorption is hindered by smoking, air
pollution, alcohol, or stress. Vitamin C is abundant in ALOE
VERA JUICE, BARLEY GRASS, CHLORELLA, GOJI BERRIES,
GREEN TEA, KIWIFRUIT, SPROUTS, and WHEATGRASS
JUICE, and is present in ARAME, ASPARAGUS, BOK CHOY,
CELERIAC, FAVA BEANS, FENNEL, FIDDLEHEAD FERNS,
GARLIC, GINGKO, KALE, KOHLRABI, LOTUS ROOT, MACA,
NETTLES, OKRA, OREGANO, PARSLEY, PLANTAINS,
POMEGRANATES, RAPINI, ROOIBOS, ROYAL JELLY, SAGE,
SARSAPARILLA, SWEETPOTATO, and SORREL.

VITAMIN E

This fat-soluble vitamin boosts the oxygen-carrying capacity of red blood cells and helps get oxygen to tissues, protects enzymes and other antioxidants, and helps make antibodies. Fats and oils that contain vitamin E are less likely to oxidize or go rancid. Get your share by eating ALOE VERA JUICE, CHLORELLA, DONG QUAI, GOJI BERRIES, GRAPESEED OIL, KIWIFRUIT, HEMP SEEDS, KAMUT, MACA, MOLASSES, NETTLES, OREGANO, ROYAL JELLY, SESAME OIL, SPROUTS, or WHEATGRASS JUICE.

CHLOROPHYLL

This plant pigment, a.k.a. "green blood," is a purifier needed to make new red blood cells and maintain ample oxygen in the bloodstream. It exists in ALFALFA, CHLORELLA, NETTLES, OREGANO, PARSLEY, ROOIBOS, SPROUTS, and WHEATGRASS JUICE.

CALCIUM

This mineral helps the kidneys do their thing, eliminates heavy metals, and regulates pH balance. The most abundant mineral in the body, calcium comprises 2-3 pounds of our body weight, although only 20-30% of the calcium we eat gets used. Its absorption can be hindered (or neutralized) by excessive protein and fat in the diet, and increased by exercise. It can be found in ALFALFA, ALOE VERA JUICE, AMARANTH, ARAME, ASAFOETIDA, BARLEY GRASS, BROWN RICE, CELERIAC, CHICK PEAS, FENNEL, GINGKO, HIJIKI, JERUSALEM ARTICHOKES, JOB'S TEARS, KALE, KIWIFRUIT, KOHLRABI, LUPINS, MACA, MOLASSES, NATTO,

OREGANO, PARSLEY, RAPINI, SAGE, SARSAPARILLA, SEI-TAN, SORREL, SPELT, SPIRULINA, SPROUTS, SWEETPO-TATO, TAHINI, TARO, TEFF, WHEATGRASS JUICE, and YERBA MATE.

IRON

Found in every cell in the body, this mineral is needed to make hemoglobin, which enables red blood cells to carry oxygen. It also helps the respiratory process. Its absorption can be hindered by coffee, tea, eggs, and sweets. Iron is available in large doses in sea vegetables like arame and hijiki, and in somewhat smaller doses in ALFALFA, ALOE VERA JUICE, AMARANTH, ASAFOETIDA, BARLEY GRASS, BLUE CORN, BROWN RICE, BURDOCK, CHICK PEAS, CHLO-RELLA, DONG QUAI, FAVA BEANS, FENNEL, GINGKO, JERUSALEM ARTICHOKES, JOB'S TEARS, KALE, LENTILS, LUPINS, MACA, MAITAKE, MILLET, MOLASSES, NATTO, OREGANO, PARSLEY, SARSAPARILLA, SPELT, SPIRULI-NA, SPROUTS, TAHINI, TARO, TEFF, and WHEATGRASS JUICE.

MAGNESIUM

Seventy percent of this mineral is found in the skeleton. Its job is to balance calcium levels, help the body utilize other antioxidants, and metabolize carbohydrates. It exists in ALFALFA, ALOE VERA JUICE, AMARANTH, CACAO, KAMUT, KIWIFRUIT, MACA, MOLASSES, OKRA, PLAN-TAINS, SORREL, and WHEATGRASS JUICE.

POTASSIUM

This mineral, the third most plentiful in the body (after calcium and phosphorus), helps detox the kidneys and maintain a balance of minerals and of pH levels. Found mostly in the cells, it works in balance with sodium found in the fluid outside the cells. It can be found in AC VINEGAR, ADUKI BEANS, ALFALFA, ALOE VERA JUICE, AMARANTH, CELE-RIAC, FAVA BEANS, FENNEL, GARLIC, HIJIKI, KIWIFRUIT, KOHLRABI, MAITAKE, MOLASSES, OREGANO, PARSLEY, PLANTAINS, RAPINI, SAGE, SARSAPARILLA, SORREL, SWEETPOTATO, WHEATGRASS JUICE, and WILD RICE.

ZINC

This trace element is used by the thymus gland to make virus-killing T cells. It is also used to make RNA and DNA, and to help the body absorb B vitamins. It also acts as a sort of "traffic policeman," directing the absorption of vitamins and overseeing enzyme systems. Zinc often gets destroyed in food processing, especially then grinding of grain into flour. Reclaim some by ingesting ALOE VERA JUICE, BLUE CORN, KAMUT, MOLASSES, OREGANO, or TVP/TSP.

ANTIOXIDANT ENZYMES

These are metabolic catalysts whose sole function is to elimi-nate free radicals. The group contains two main members, superoxide dismutase (SOD) and catalase (CAT), and eight secondary members, each designed to deactivate a specific type of free radical. Unlike a vitamin molecule, which attacks a single free radical, an antioxidant enzyme molecule can conquer thousands. Get your supply from ALFALFA, SHII-TAKE, SPROUTS, or WHEATGRASS JUICE.

VITAMIN D

This is not really a vitamin but a hormone made by the body. Sunlight landing on the skin converts a chemical called "ergosterol" into vitamin D, also known as the "sunshine vitamin." Interestingly, darker skin produces less vitamin D than lighter skin. Foods containing vitamin A usually contain some "provitamin D."

PHOSPHORUS

This is the body's second most abundant mineral, making up about 1% of our weight, 90% of which resides in our bones and teeth as phosphates (phosphorus + oxygen). Its absorption is dependent on vitamin D and calcium. Modern humans tend to get too much phosphorus vs. calcium, as most (non-organic) veggies are fed with phosphate fertilizers. Phosphates are also often added to processed foods to give them an acid flavor. Sources of phosphorus include ALFALFA, ASAFOETIDA, CHICK PEAS, HEMP SEEDS, HIJIKI, JERUSALEM ARTICHOKES, LENTILS, MACA, MAITAKE, MOLASSES, NATTO, SORREL, TARO, WILD RICE, and YERBA MATE.

IODINE

is needed to make thyroxine, which helps regulate the body's energy. Too little of this trace element during pregancy can cause cretinism and, at other times, lead to an enlarged thyroid, or goiter. Iodine is abundant in sea vegetables like ARAME, HIJIKI, AND KOMBU.

ANTI-CANCER

The following foods have been shown to inhibit the growth of cancerous cells or contain chemicals which produce such effects: ASPARAGUS ROOT, BURDOCK, BOK CHOY, BOSWELLIA, BROCCOLI SPROUTS, CHLORELLA, FLAX SEED, GARLIC, PAU D'ARCO, REISHI, MISO, QUINOA, and WILD CELERY SEEDS.

ANTI-CHOLESTEROL/HYPERTENSION

The following foods are known to lower cholesterol or high blood pressure or otherwise help circulation: BARLEY, CHLORELLA, GARLIC, GOTU KOLA, GREEN TEA, JERUSALEM ARTICHOKES, LICORICE ROOT, MA HUANG, MISO, NONI, PSYLLIUM, PRIMROSE OIL, REISHI, SHIITAKE, SUMA, QUINOA, WILD CELERY SEEDS, YAMABUSHITAKE, and YARROW.

ANTI-AGING

These foods are believed to promote longevity: AC VINEGAR, BOSWELLIA, CHLORELLA, FO-TI and ROYAL JELLY.

DIGESTION/ALKALINITY

The following foods are often consumed to cure indigestion or to balance the body's pH level and combat acidity and heartburn: ACIDOPHILUS, ADUKI BEANS, APPLE CIDER VINEGAR, BARLEY GRASS, BURDOCK, CAYENNE, FENNEL, GALANGAL ROOT, GREEN TEA, KOMBUCHA, KUZU, JERUSALEM ARTICHOKES, MILLET, NONI, PSYLLIUM, SHIITAKE, TARO, and UMEBOSHI.

BRAIN BOOSTING

These plants are thought to improve memory and mental functioning: CACAO, GINGKO, GOTU KOLA, FAVA BEANS, and YAMABUSHITAKE.

GENERAL HEALING

The following foods are reported to impart vim and vigor or have curative powers: APPLE CIDER VINEGAR, ALOE VERA JUICE, ASHWAGANDA, ASTRAGALUS, BAMBOO MANNA, BHRINGARAJ, BURDOCK, BLUE CORN, COLOS-TRUM, CAT'S CLAW, FLAX SEED, GINGER, GINSENG, GOJI BERRIES, GRAPESEED, HOLY BASIL, LICORICE ROOT, LUPINS, NONI, PAO D'ARCO, PRIMROSE OIL, ST. JOHN'S WORT, SCHIZANDRA, REISHI, TEA TREE OIL, THYME, TURMERIC, WINGED BEANS, and YARROW.

· All excess energy in the body is stored as fat.

· Just as carbohydrates are made from sugars, and protein from amino acids, fat is composed of fatty acids and a chemical called glycerol.

· Saturated fats are solid at room temperature, while unsaturated fats are liquids (oils).

· Cholesterol is a kind of lipid that is produced in ample amounts by the body itself, which means it doesn't need to be obtained from other sources. Plants do not contain cholesterol, while all animal foods do. Excess cholesterol can harden and clog arteries.

ESSENTIAL FATTY ACIDS (EFAS)

To find out about essential fatty acids, see FLAX SEED and HEMP SEEDS. Foods containing these vital substances include ACAI, BURDOCK, FLAX SEEDS, HEMP SEEDS, GRAPESEED OIL, PRIMROSE OIL, SESAME OIL, and SPIRULINA.

PROTEIN

Of all the nutrients in our diet, protein is the least likely to be deficient. Modern nutritionists, in fact, say that any diet other than one of pure junk food contains ample protein, and that most folks (even some vegetarians) get too much of the stuff. Excessive protein has been linked to diseases like osteoporosis, as protein sucks calcium right out of the bones.

Protein is composed of various combinations of 22 amino acids, all but 8 of which can produced by the body. These elusive 8, which must be obtained from food, have been dubbed "the essentials," and protein that contains all of them is a "complete" protein. Not many foods contain complete proteins, but, fortunately, foods that are low in certain aminos can be combined with foods high in those aminos (but perhaps low in others) to boost the usable protein content. This "complementary protein" action happens, for example, in the globally popular bean-with-grain combo, such as frijoles with tortillas, chapati with lentils, couscous with chick peas, and tofu or tempeh with rice.

Protein is abundant in TVP/TSP (up to 70%), SPIRULINA (65%), CHLORELLA (60%), ROYAL JELLY (35%), HEMP SEEDS (25%), SEITAN, and soy products like tofu (30%), TEMPEH (19.5%) and MISO. It's available in legumes like CHICK PEAS, FAVA BEANS, LENTILS, LUPINS, and WINGED BEANS; grains like ALFALFA, AMARANTH, BROWN RICE, BUCKWHEAT, JOB'S TEARS, KAMUT, MILLET, SORGHUM, SPELT, TEFF, TRITICALE, and QUINOA; veggies like ARAME, JERUSALEM ARTICHOKE, KALE, MACA, MAITAKE, REISHI, and SHIITAKE; and other foods like BARLEY GRASS, BREWER'S YEAST, GOJI BERRIES, NATTO, SPROUTS, TAHINI, WHEATGRASS JUICE, and WILD RICE.

Sugar is essential for life; added sugar is not. Despite this, the typical American gets from 25 to 40% of his or her daily calories from sugar, which adds up to about 35 teaspoons per day or 127 pounds per year. White or table sugar in particular, containing empty calories with no nutrition, tends to make us obese. It's also heavily processed, being the second least energy-efficient food after meat. This section gives a short sugar synopsis followed by a list of alternatives to white sugar, some healthy, some not.

COMPLEX CARBOHYDRATES

are made of many sugar units joined together, which digestive enzymes gradually break down into glucose that is introduced steadily into the bloodstream. They are found in grains, beans, friuts, and vegetables

SIMPLE SUGARS

enter the bloodstream directly, causing a sudden rise in blood sugar and stimulating the release of insulin in the body, resulting in a corresponding drop in blood sugar levels (a "sugar low"). The most common simple sugars are:

GLUCOSE

One of the simplest sugars; also called blood sugar or dextrose.

FRUCTOSE

is found in fruits and vegetable. It metabolizes slightly more slowly than sucrose

SUCROSE

is a mix of glucose and fructose.

MALTOSE

is freed by the digestion of starch. It consists of two glucose molecules.

AGAVE NECTAR

is usually derived from the same cactus-like plant used to make tequila. Although sweeter than honey or sugar, it is low in glucose.

AMASAKE

is a thick liquid made from sweet brown rice and koji (a mold used in miso, tamari, and soy).

BARLEY MALT & RICE SYRUP

are made by cooking whole grains. They contain protein and minerals, and their sugars (maltose and others) are released slowly into the bloodstream.

BEET SUGARS

are extracted from sugar beets. The production process is similar to that of cane sugars.

BROWN & TURBINADO SUGARS

are by-products from the making of refined sugar from cane. Both contain at least 95% glucose and have no nutritional value. The former is often white sugar with molasses re-added.

FRUIT JUICE CONCENTRATES,

usually made from pineapples, white grapes, or dates, are comprised mostly of fructose.

HONEY

contains some minerals and B vitamins. Raw honey retains the pollen.

MAPLE SYRUP

is mostly glucose and water, with trace amounts of iron, calcium, potassium, and phosphorus.

MOLASSES.

also a white sugar by-product, contains E and B vitamins, calcium, and other trace minerals.

RAW SUGAR

("Sugar in the Raw") is vegan cane sugar not subjected to the final refining steps, which often involve filtration through charred animal bone.

STEVIA & LICORICE ROOT

are sweet herbs that have the added benefit of being safe for diabetics.

SUCANAT

(SUgar CAne NATural) is the dehydrated juice of organic sugar cane (it's sometimes called dehydrated cane juice or granulated cane juice). It's composed of 84% sucrose, 7% fructose, 5% glucose, 1% minerals (including sodium, potassium, calcium, and magnesium), and trace vitamins.

YACON

is made from a South American plant whose tubers and leaves contain inulin, which maintains blood sugar levels while being beneficial for digestion and immune health.

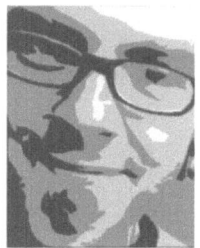

Darrin Drda is a writer, illustrator, designer, musician, cartoonist, and peacenik who was born, raised, and educated in Illinois. He holds an MA in Philosophy, Cosmology and Consciousness from the California Institute of Integral Studies in San Francisco, where he now lives with his wife, Annabelle.

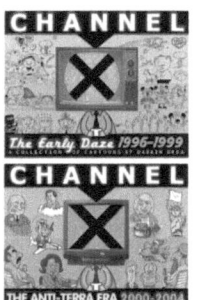

Darrin's other self-published works include two compilations of his long-running comic, "Channel X," which can be found at the following URLs:

Channel X: The Early Daze
https://www.createspace.com/3388868
Channel X: The Anti-Terra Era
https://www.createspace.com/3389907

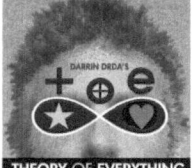

Also available are the following CDs, recorded with Darrin's former band, Theory of Everything.

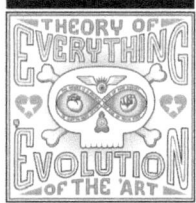

Darrin Drda's Theory of Everything:
https://www.createspace.com/1766472
'Evolution of the 'Art:
https://www.createspace.com/1766487
Loveway:
https://www.createspace.com/1766453

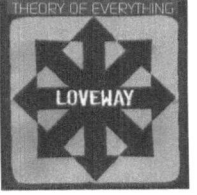

For more information and AV stimulation, please visit www.darrindrda.org. Darrin can be reached at darrindrda@gmail.com.